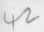

THE KING'S SPEECH

THE KING'S SPEECH

How One Man Saved the British Monarchy

Mark Logue
and Peter Conradi

WINDSOR
PARAGON

First published 2010
by Quercus
This Large Print edition published 2011
by AudioGO Ltd
by arrangement with
Quercus

Hardcover ISBN: 978 1 445 85914 9
Softcover   ISBN: 978 1 445 85915 6

British Library Cataloguing in Publication Data available

Printed and bound in Great Britain by
MPG Books Group Limited

Contents

PICTURE CREDITS

All images courtesy Logue family archive except

Acknowledgments

Firstly, I owe an enormous debt of gratitude to Peter Conradi. If it wasn't for his unflinching determination in the face of a daunting schedule, this book may never have existed.

I would like to thank my extended family, especially Alex Marshall, whose discovery of a treasure trove of letters led to a more profound understanding of Lionel's life and work. Anne Logue for her recollections, Sarah Logue for her time and Patrick and Nickie Logue for their help in looking after the archive. Also my lovely wife Ruth and our children for allowing this project to take over our lives for a year. Without their support this book would never have happened.

Thanks also to Caroline Bowen for answering so many questions about speech therapy, and who was pivotal in putting the film's producers in touch with the Logue family, and starting the ball rolling. Francesca Budd for her help in transcribing the archive and her support throughout the filming process. All involved in the film, Tom Hooper, David Seidler, Colin Firth, Geoffrey Rush and everyone at See-Saw Films, especially Iain Canning.

Jenny Savill at Andrew Nurnberg Associates was central in getting the book published. I also give my warm thanks to Richard Milner and Joshua Ireland at Quercus, without whom this book would not have got off the ground.

I'd also like to thank Meredith Hooper for some

illuminating facts, Michael Thornton for letting us publish his accounts of Evelyn Laye, Neil Urbino, whose genealogy work helped dig deeper, Marista Leishman for her help with the Reith diaries, and David J Radcliffe for his own account of his fight with a stammer.

Margaret Hosking and The University of Adelaide and Susanne Dowling at Murdoch University were an enormous help in digging out library material.

Thanks also to Tony Aldous, school archivist at Prince Alfred College, Peta Madalena, archivist at Scotch College and Lyn Williams at Lion Nathan. The Royal College of Speech and Language Therapists were extremely helpful, especially Robin Matheou.

Finally, thanks to the National Library of Australia, the State Library of South Australia and the State Library of Western Australia, the Australian Dictionary of Biography and the National Portrait Gallery, London.

Mark Logue

Introduction

When I was growing up in the 1970s and 1980s we lived in Belgium, where my father, Antony, worked as a lawyer at the European headquarters of Procter & Gamble. Over the years we moved between various houses on the outskirts of Brussels, but there was one constant: regardless of where we were, a collection of photographs and mementos would be set up on a mantelpiece or windowsill.

Among them was a photograph of my father in his Scots Guards uniform; another of him and my mother, Elizabeth, on their wedding day in 1953, and a picture of my Australian-born paternal grandfather, Lionel, and his wife, Myrtle. Also, more intriguingly, there was a leather-framed portrait of King George VI, the father of the present Queen, signed and dated 12 May 1937, the day of his coronation; another picture of him and his wife, Elizabeth, better known to my generation as the Queen Mother, and their two daughters, the future Queen Elizabeth, then a girl of eleven, and her little sister, Margaret Rose; and a third of the royal couple, dated 1928, when they were still the Duke and Duchess of York, signed Elizabeth and Albert.

The significance of all these photographs must have been explained to me, but as a young boy I never paid too much attention. I understood the link with royalty was through Lionel, but he was ancient history to me; he had died in 1953, twelve years before I was born. The sum of my knowledge about my grandfather was that he had been the King's speech therapist—whatever that was—and I left it at that. I never asked any more questions and no more detailed information was volunteered. I was far more interested in the various medals and buttons laid out alongside the photographs. I used particularly to enjoy dressing up in my father's officer's belt and hat, and playing at soldiers with the medals pinned proudly on my shirt.

But as I grew older, and had children of my own, I began to wonder about who my ancestors were and where they had come from. The growing general interest in genealogy further piqued my curiosity. Looking back through the family tree, I came across a great-grandmother from Melbourne who had fourteen children, only seven of whom survived beyond infancy. I also learnt that my great-great-grandfather left Ireland for Australia in 1850 aboard the SS *Boyne*.

As far as I was concerned, my grandfather was only one among many members of an extended family divided between Australia, Ireland and Britain. That remained the case even after the death of my father in 2001, when I was left the task of going through the personal papers he had kept in a tall grey filing cabinet. There, among the wills, deeds and other important documents, were hundreds of old letters and photographs collected by my grandfather—all neatly filed away in chronological order in a document wallet.

It was only in June 2009, when I was approached by Iain Canning, who was producing a film, *The King's Speech*, about Lionel, that I began to understand the significance of the role played by my grandfather: about how he had helped the then Duke of York, who reluctantly became King in December 1936 after the abdication of his elder brother, Edward VIII, in his lifelong battle against a chronic stammer that turned every public speech or radio broadcast into a terrifying ordeal. I began to appreciate that his life and work could be of interest to a far wider audience beyond my own family.

That April, Lionel had been the subject of the Afternoon Play on BBC Radio 4, again called *A King's Speech*, by Mark Burgess. This film was to be something far bigger, however—a major motion picture, with a big-name cast that included Helena Bonham Carter, Colin Firth, Geoffrey Rush, Michael Gambon and Derek Jacobi. It is directed by Tom Hooper, the man behind the acclaimed *The Damned United*, which showed a very different side of recent English history: the football manager Brian Clough's short and stormy tenure as manager of Leeds United in 1974.

Canning and Hooper, of course, wanted their film to be as historically accurate as possible, so I set out to try and discover as much as I could about my grandfather. The obvious starting point was my father's filing cabinet: examining Lionel's papers properly for the first time, I found vividly written diaries in which he had recorded his meetings with the King in extraordinary detail. There was copious correspondence, often warm and friendly, with George VI himself, and various other records—including a little appointment card, covered in my grandfather's spider-like handwriting, in which he described his first encounter with the future King in his small consulting room in Harley Street on 19 October 1926.

Taken together with other fragments of information I managed to gather online, and the few pages of references to Lionel included in most biographies of George VI, this allowed me to learn more about my grandfather's unique relationship with the King and also to correct some of the part-truths and overstretched memories that had become blurred across the generations.

It soon became clear, however, that the archive was incomplete. Missing were a number of letters and diary entries from the 1920s and 1930s, snippets of which had been quoted in John Wheeler Bennett's authorized biography of George VI, published in 1958. Also nowhere to be found were the scrapbooks of newspaper cuttings that, as I knew from my cousins, Lionel had collected for much of his adult life.

Perhaps the most disappointing absence, though, was that of a letter, written by the King in December 1944, which had particularly captured my imagination. Its existence was revealed in a passage in Lionel's diary in which he described a conversation between the two men after the monarch had delivered his annual Christmas message to the nation for the first time without my grandfather at his side.

'My job is over, Sir,' Lionel told him.

'Not at all,' the King replied. 'It is the preliminary work that counts, and that is where you are indispensable.' Then, according to Lionel's account, 'he thanked me, and two days later wrote me a very beautiful letter, which I hope will be treasured by my descendants'.

Had I had the letter I would have treasured it, but it was nowhere to be found amid the mass of correspondence, newspaper cuttings and diary entries. This missing letter inspired me to leave no stone unturned, to exhaust every line of enquiry in what became a quest to piece together as many details as I could of my grandfather's life. I pestered relatives, returning to speak to them time and again. I wrote to Buckingham Palace, to the Royal Archives at Windsor Castle and to the authors and publishers of books about George VI, in the hope that the letter may have been among material they had borrowed from my father or his two elder brothers, and had failed to return. But there was no trace of it.

Towards the end of 2009 I was invited on to the set of *The King's Speech* during filming in Portland Place, in London. During a break I met Geoffrey Rush, who plays my grandfather, and Ben Wimsett, who portrays my father aged ten. After getting over the initial strangeness of seeing someone as a child I'd only ever known as a man, I became fascinated by a scene in which Rush's character hovers over my father and his elder brother, Valentine, played by Dominic Applewhite, while they are made to recite Shakespeare. It reminded me of a similar real-life scene when I was a boy and my father obliged me to do the same.

My father had a passion—and a gift—for poetry and verse, often repeating verbatim entire passages that he remembered since childhood. He used to revel in his ability to rattle off reams of Hilaire Belloc as a party piece to guests. But it was from my elder sister, Sarah, that he derived the most satisfaction: indeed, she was often moved to tears by his recitals.

At the time, I don't remember being much impressed by my father's talent. Looking back on the scene as an adult, however, I can appreciate both his perseverance and the acute frustration he must have felt at my reluctance to share the love of poetry that his father had instilled in him.

Filming ended in January 2010, and this also marked the beginning of a more personal voyage of discovery for me. Canning and Hooper did not set out to make a documentary but rather a biopic, which, although true to the spirit of my grandfather, concentrates on a narrow period of time: from the first meeting between my grandfather and the future King in 1926 until the outbreak of war in 1939.

Inspired by the film, I wanted to tell the complete story of my grandfather's life, from his childhood in Adelaide, South Australia, in the 1880s right the way through to his death. Thus I started extensive and detailed research into his character and what he had done during his life. It was in many ways a frustrating process because, despite Lionel's professional status, very little was known about the methods he employed with the King. Although he wrote a few articles for the press about the treatment of stammering and other speech impediments, he never set out his methods in a formal way and had no student or apprentice with whom to share the secrets of his work. Nor—probably because of the discretion with which he always treated his relationship with the King—did he write up his most famous case.

Then, in July 2010, with the publishers pressing

for the manuscript, my perseverance finally paid off. On hearing of my quest for material, my cousin, Alex Marshall, contacted me to say that she had found some boxes of documents relating to my grandfather. She didn't think they would be of much use but, even so, I invited myself up to her home in Rutland to take a look. I was greeted with several volumes arranged on a table in her dining room: there were two Bankers Boxes full of correspondence between the King and Lionel dating from 1926 to 1952 and two more boxes filled with manuscripts and press cuttings, which Lionel had carefully glued into two big scrapbooks, one green and the other blue.

To my delight, Alex also had the missing parts of the archive, together with three volumes of letters and a section of diary that my grandmother, Myrtle, kept when she and my grandfather embarked on a trip round the world in 1910, and also during the first few months of the Second World War. Written in a more personal style than Lionel's diary, this gave a far more revealing insight into the minutiae of their life together. The documents, running to hundreds of pages, were a fascinating treasure trove that I spent days going through and deciphering; my only regret was that the letter that I had been so desperate to find was not among them.

It is all this material that forms the basis for this book, which Peter Conradi, an author and journalist with *The Sunday Times*, has helped me to put together. I hope that in reading it, you will come to share my fascination with my grandfather and his unique and very close relationship with King George VI.

Although I have endeavoured to research my grandfather's life exhaustively, there may be pieces of information about him that still remain undiscovered. If you are related to Lionel Logue, were a patient or colleague of his, or if you have any other information about him and his work, I would love to hear from you. I can be contacted on lionellogue@gmail.com

Mark Logue
London, August 2010

CHAPTER ONE

God Save the King

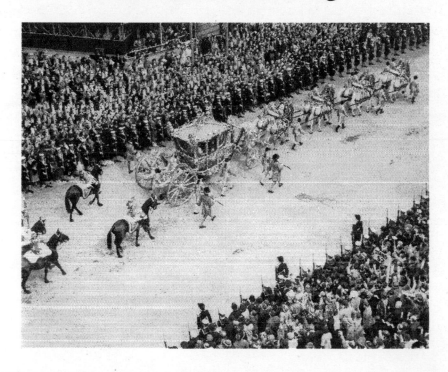

The royal party on their way to the coronation of
George VI

Albert Frederick Arthur George, King of the United Kingdom and the British Dominions and the last Emperor of India, woke up with a start. It was just after 3 a.m. The bedroom in Buckingham Palace he had occupied since becoming monarch five months earlier was normally a haven of peace and quiet in the heart of London, but on this particular morning his slumbers had been rudely interrupted by the crackle of loudspeakers being tested outside on Constitution Hill. 'One of them might have been in our room,' he wrote in his diary.[1] And then, just when he thought he might finally be able to go back to sleep, the marching bands and troops started up.

It was 12 May 1937, and the forty-one-year-old King was about to face one of the greatest—and most nerve-racking—days of his life: his coronation. Traditionally, the ceremony is held eighteen months after the monarch comes to the throne, leaving time not just for all the preparations but also for a decent period of mourning for the previous king or queen. This coronation was different: the date had already been chosen to crown his elder brother, who had become king on the death of their father, George V, in January 1936. Edward VIII had lasted less than a year on the throne, however, after succumbing to the charms of Wallis Simpson, an American divorcee, and it was his younger brother, Albert, Duke of York, who reluctantly succeeded him when he abdicated that December. Albert took the name George VI—as both a tribute to his late father and a sign of continuity with his reign

3

after the upheavals of the previous year that had plunged the British monarchy into one of the greatest crises in its history.

At about the same time, in the considerably less grand setting of Sydenham Hill, in the suburbs of south-east London, a handsome man in his late fifties, with a shock of brown hair and bright blue eyes, was also stirring. He, too, had a big day ahead of him. The Australian-born son of a publican, his name was Lionel Logue and since his first meeting with the future monarch just over a decade earlier, he had occupied a curious but increasingly influential role at the heart of the royal family.

Just to be on the safe side, Logue (who was a reluctant driver) had had a chauffeur sleep overnight at his house. With his statuesque wife Myrtle, who was to accompany him on that momentous day, he began to prepare himself for the journey into town. Myrtle, who was wearing £5,000 worth of jewellery, looked radiant. A meeting with a hairdresser whom they'd agreed to pick up along the way would add the final touch. Logue, in full court costume, was rather conscious of his silk-stockinged legs and had to keep taking care not to trip over his sword.

As the hours ticked by and the streets of London began to fill with crowds of well-wishers, many of whom had slept out on camp beds, both men's sense of apprehension grew. The King had a 'sinking feeling inside' and could eat no breakfast. 'I knew that I was to spend a most trying day & to go through the most important ceremony in my life,' he wrote in his diary that evening. 'The hours of waiting before leaving for Westminster Abbey

4

were the most nerve racking.'[2]

With origins dating back almost a millennium, the coronation of a British monarch in Westminster Abbey is a piece of national pageantry unmatched anywhere in the world. At the centre of the ceremony is the anointing: while the monarch is seated in the medieval King Edward's Chair, a canopy over his head, the Archbishop of Canterbury touches his hands, breast and head with consecrated oil. A cocktail of orange, roses, cinnamon, musk and ambergris, it is dispensed from a filigreed spoon filled from an eagle-shaped ampulla. By that act, the monarch is consecrated before God to the service of his peoples to whom he has sworn a grave oath. For a man as deeply religious as King George VI, it was difficult to overestimate the significance of this avowal of his dependence on the Almighty for the spirit, strength and power needed to do right by his subjects.

To be at the centre of such a ceremony—all the while balancing an ancient 7lb crown on his head—would have been a huge ordeal for anyone, but the King had particular reason to view what was in store for him with trepidation: plagued since childhood with a series of medical ailments, he also suffered from a debilitating stammer. Embarrassing enough in small gatherings, it turned public speaking into a major ordeal. The King, in the words of America's *Time* magazine, was the 'most famed contemporary stammerer' in the world,[3] joining a roll call of prominent names stretching back to antiquity that included Aesop, Aristotle, Demosthenes, Virgil, Erasmus and Darwin.

5

Worse, in the weeks running up to the coronation, the King had been forced to endure a whispering campaign about his health, stirred up by supporters of his embittered elder brother, who was now living in exile in France. The new King, it was rumoured, was in such a poor physical state that he would not be able to endure the coronation ceremony, let alone discharge his functions as sovereign. Further fuel for the campaign had been provided by the King's decision not to go ahead with an Accession Durbar in Delhi that his predecessor had agreed should take place during the cold-weather season of 1937–8.

The invited congregation had to be in the Abbey by around 7 a.m. Crowds cheered them as they passed; a special Tube train running from Kensington High Street to Westminster was laid on for Members of the House of Commons and for peers and peeresses, who travelled in full robes and wearing their coronets.

Logue and his wife set off from their home at 6.40, travelling through deserted streets, northwards through Denmark Hill and Camberwell Green and then westwards towards the newly rebuilt Chelsea Bridge, which had been opened less than a week earlier by William Lyon Mackenzie King, the Canadian prime minister who was in town for the coronation. One by one, the police constables spotted the 'P' in green lettering on the windscreen of their car and waved them through, until, just before the Tate Gallery, they ran into a jam of cars from all over London converging on the Abbey. They got out as they reached the covered way opposite the statue of Richard the Lionheart in Parliament Square and had squeezed into their seats by 7.30.

The King and Queen travelled to the Abbey in the Gold State Coach, a magnificent enclosed carriage drawn by eight horses that had been first used by King George III to open parliament in 1762. For the present King, the presence of his wife, Queen Elizabeth, was an enormous reassurance. During their fourteen years of marriage, she had been a hugely calming influence on him; whenever he faltered in the middle of a speech, she would squeeze his arm affectionately, willing him to go on—usually with success.

Seated in the royal box were the King's mother, Queen Mary, and his two young daughters. The smaller one, Princess Margaret Rose, now aged six and naughty at the best of times, was bored and squirming. As the interminably long service continued, she stuck her finger in her eye, pulled her ears, swung her legs, rested her head on her elbow and tickled her rather more serious elder sister, Elizabeth, who had recently celebrated her eleventh birthday. As was so often the case, the elder girl found herself urging her sister to be good. Queen Mary finally quietened Margaret Rose by giving her a pair of opera glasses to peek through.

Reassurance of another kind was provided by Logue, whose presence in a box overlooking the ceremony was a sign of his importance to the King. A self-described 'common colonial', who despite a career devoted to elocution had never quite succeeded in shaking off his Australian accent, Logue seemed strangely out of place among the upper echelons of the British aristocracy given pride of place in the Abbey.

7

Yet it would be difficult to exaggerate the contribution to the day's momentous events that had been made by a man whom the newspapers called the King's 'speech doctor' or 'speech specialist'. Such was Logue's status that he had just been made a member of the Royal Victorian Order, an appointment entirely in the gift of the sovereign. The award was front-page news: his was, declared the *Daily Express*, 'one of the most interesting of the names in the Coronation Honours List'. Logue wore the medal proudly on his chest in the Abbey.

In the eleven years since his arrival on the boat from Australia, Logue, from his rented room in Harley Street, in the heart of the British medical establishment, had become one of the most prominent figures in the emerging field of speech therapy. For much of that time he had been helping the then Duke of York tackle his speech impediment.

For the past month they had been preparing for the great day, rehearsing over and over again the time-honoured responses that the King would have to give in the Abbey. In the years they had worked together, whether at Logue's little surgery, at Sandringham, Windsor or Buckingham Palace, they had developed a system. First Logue would study the text, spotting any words that might trip the King up, such as those that began with a hard 'k' or 'g' sound or perhaps with repeated consonants, and wherever possible, replace them with something else. Logue would then mark up the text with suggested breathing points, and the King would start practising, again and again, until he got it right—often becoming extremely

8

frustrated in the process.

But there could be no tampering with the words of the coronation service. This was the real test—and it was about to begin.

*   *   *

The various princes and princesses, both British and foreign, had started to be shown to their places at 10.15 a.m. Then came the King's mother, walking to the stately music of the official Coronation March, followed by the various state representations and then the Queen, her marvellous train carried by her six ladies-in-waiting.

'A fanfare of trumpets, and the King's procession was soon advancing, a blaze of gold and crimson,' wrote Logue in the diary in which he was to record much of his life in Britain. 'And at the end the man whom I had served for 10 years, with all my heart and soul comes, as he advances slowly towards us, looking rather pale, but every inch a King. My heart creeps up into my throat, as I realise that this man whom I serve, is to be made King of England.'

As Cosmo Lang, the Archbishop of Canterbury, led the coronation service, Logue was listening probably more intently than anyone else present in the Abbey, even though the toothache from which he was suffering kept threatening to distract him. The King seemed nervous to him at the beginning, and Logue's heart missed a beat when he started the oath, but on the whole he spoke well. When it was all over, Logue was jubilant: 'The King spoke with a beautiful inflexion,' he told a journalist.

In fact, given the pressure the King was under, it

was a wonder he had spoken his words so clearly: while holding the book with the form of service for him to read, the Archbishop had inadvertently covered the words of the Oath with his thumb. Nor was that the only mishap: when the Lord Great Chamberlain started to dress the King in his robes, his hands were shaking so much he nearly put the hilt of the sword under the King's chin rather than attaching it to the belt, where it should have been. And then, as the King sat up from the Coronation Chair, a bishop trod on his robe, almost causing him to fall over until the King ordered him pretty sharply to get off it.

Such hitches were an inevitable accompaniment to a British coronation; one of the King's main preoccupations was that Lang wouldn't put the crown on back to front, as had happened in the past, and so he had arranged that a small line of thin red cotton be inserted under one of the principal jewels at the front. Some over-zealous person had obviously removed it in the meantime, and the King was never quite sure it was the right way round. Coronations of earlier monarchs had bordered on farce: George III's in 1761 was held up for three hours after the sword of state went missing, while his son and successor George IV's was overshadowed by his row with his estranged and hated wife, Caroline of Brunswick, who had to be forcibly prevented from entering the Abbey.

None of these current minor hitches was noticed by the congregation, let alone by the thousands of people who were still lining the streets of London despite the worsening weather. When the service was over, the King and Queen took the Gold Coach by the long route back to Buckingham

Palace. By now it was pouring with rain, but this did not seem to deter the crowd who cheered them enthusiastically as they drove past. Logue and Myrtle were relaxing, eating sandwiches and the chocolate they had brought with them when, at 3.30, an amplified voice announced: 'Those in block J can proceed to the cars.' They then passed down to the entrance and another thirty minutes later their car was called and they fell into it, Logue almost tripping over that sword. They crossed back over Westminster Bridge, past the now deserted viewing stands, and reached home by 4.30. Now suffering from a headache as well as toothache, Logue took to his bed for a nap.

*   *   *

However momentous, the coronation was only part of what the King faced that day. At eight that evening he was to face an even greater ordeal: a live radio address to be broadcast to the people of the United Kingdom and her vast Empire—and again Logue was to be at his side. The speech was due to last only a few minutes, but it was no less nerve-racking for that. Over the years, the King had developed a particular terror of the microphone, which made a radio address seem even more of a challenge than a speech to a live audience. Nor was Sir John Reith, the director-general of the British Broadcasting Corporation, which had been created by Royal Charter a decade earlier, making things easier for him: he insisted that the King should broadcast live.

For weeks running up to the broadcast, Logue had been working with the King on the text. After

11

decidedly mixed rehearsals, the two men seemed confident enough—but they were not taking any chances. Over the previous few days, Robert Wood, one of the BBC's most experienced sound engineers and an expert at the emerging art of the outside broadcast, had made recordings of their various practice sessions on gramophone records, including a specially edited one that combined all the best passages in one. Even so, Logue was still feeling nervous as a car brought him back to the Palace at 7 p.m.

When he arrived he joined Alexander Hardinge, the King's private secretary, and Reith for a whisky and soda. As the three men stood drinking, word came down from upstairs that the King was ready for Logue. To the Australian's eye, the King looked in good shape, despite what had already been an extremely emotional day. They went through the speech once at the microphone and then returned to his room, where they were joined by the Queen, who looked tired but happy.

Logue could sense the King's nerves, however, and to take his mind off the ordeal ahead, Logue kept him chatting about the events of the day right up until the moment just after eight o'clock when the opening notes of the National Anthem came through the loudspeakers.

'Good Luck, Bertie,' said the Queen as her husband walked up to the microphone.

'It is with a very full heart I speak to you tonight,' the King began, his words relayed by the BBC not just to his subjects in Britain but to those in the farflung Empire, including Logue's homeland. 'Never before has a newly crowned King been able to talk to all his peoples in their own homes on the day of his coronation . . .'

Perspiration was running down Logue's back.

'The Queen and I wish health and happiness to you all, and we do not forget at this time of celebration those who are living under the shadow of sickness,' the King continued, 'beautifully', as Logue thought.

'I cannot find words with which to thank you for your love and loyalty to the Queen and myself . . . I will only say this: that if in the coming years I can show my gratitude in service to you, that is the way above all others that I should choose . . . The Queen and I will always keep in our hearts the inspiration of this day. May we ever be worthy of the goodwill which I am proud to think surrounds us at the outset of my reign. I thank you from my heart, and may God bless you all.'

By the time the speech was over, Logue was so worked up he couldn't talk. The King handed Wood his Coronation Medal and, shortly afterwards, the Queen joined them. 'It was wonderful, Bertie, much better than the record,' she told him.

The King bade farewell to Wood and, turning to Logue, pressed his hand as he said, 'Good night, Logue, I thank you very much.' The Queen did the same, her blue eyes shining as, overcome by the occasion, he replied, 'The greatest thing in my life, your Majesty, is being able to serve you.'

'Good night. Thank you,' she repeated, before adding softly, 'God bless you.'

Tears began to well in Logue's eyes, and he felt like a fool as he went downstairs to Hardinge's room, where he had another whisky and soda and immediately regretted it. It was, he reflected later,

13

a silly thing to do on an empty stomach, as the whole world began to spin around and his speech to slur. He nevertheless set off with Hardinge in the car, dropping him off at St James's before turning south-east towards home. As he looked back over the momentous events of the day, Logue's mind kept turning to the moment when the Queen had said to him 'God bless you'—that, and how he really ought to get his tooth fixed.

Logue spent the next day almost entirely in bed, ignoring the insistent ring of the telephone as his friends called to pass on their congratulations. The newspapers' verdict on the speech was overwhelmingly positive. 'The King's voice last night was strong and deep, resembling to a startling degree the voice of his father,' reported the *Star*. 'His words came through firmly, clearly— and without hesitation.' Both men couldn't have wished for a better accolade.

CHAPTER TWO

The 'common colonial'

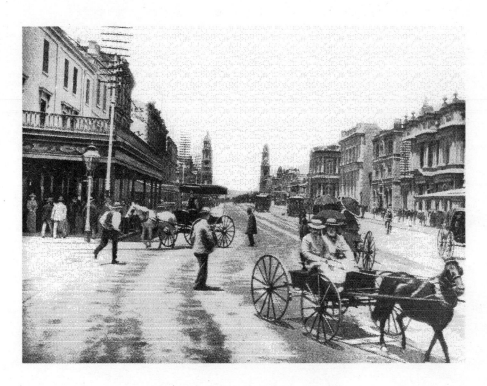

Adelaide in the 1880s

Adelaide in the 1880s was a city overflowing with civic pride. Named in honour of Queen Adelaide, the German-born consort of King William IV, it had been founded in 1836 as the planned capital of a freely settled British province in Australia. It was laid out in a grid pattern, interspaced by wide boulevards and large public squares, and surrounded by parkland. By the time of its half centenary, it had become a comfortable place to live: from 1860 residents had been able to enjoy water piped in from the Thorndon Park reservoir, horse-drawn trams and railways made it easy to move around, and by night the streets were lit by gas lights. In 1874 it acquired a university; seven years later, the South Australian Art Gallery opened its doors for the first time.

It was here, close to College Town on the outskirts of the city, that Lionel George Logue was born on 26 February 1880, the eldest of four children. His grandfather, Edward Logue, originally a Dubliner, had arrived in 1850 and set up Logue's Brewery on King William Street. The city at this time had dozens of independent breweries, but Edward Logue's did especially well; the *Adelaide Observer* attributed its success to the good water and the 'more than ordinary skill' of the proprietor, who was able to produce 'ale of a character which enables him to compete successfully with all other manufacturers of the nut brown creature comfort'.

Logue never knew his grandfather; Edward died in 1868, and his brewery was taken over by his widow Sarah, and her business partner Edwin

17

Smith, who later bought her out. After several mergers, the original business was eventually to become part of the South Australian Brewing Company.

Logue's father George, who was born in 1856 in Adelaide, was educated at St Peter's College and, after leaving school, went to work at the brewery, rising to the position of accountant. He later became licensee of the Burnside Hotel, which he ran together with his wife Lavinia, and then took over the Elephant and Castle Hotel, which still stands today on West Terrace. It was, Logue recalled, a perfect childhood. 'I had a wonderfully happy home, as we were a very united family.'

Logue was sent to school at Prince Alfred College, one of Adelaide's oldest boys' schools and arch rival of St Peter's. The school enjoyed considerable success both academically and in sports, especially cricket and Australian Rules Football. By his own admission, however, Logue struggled to find an academic subject at which he excelled. His epiphany came unexpectedly: kept back for detention one day, he opened a book at random: it was Longfellow's *The Song of Hiawatha*. The words seemed to leap out of the page at him:

> Then Iagoo, the great boaster,
> He the marvellous story-teller,
> He the traveller and the talker,
> He the friend of old Nokomis,
> Made a bow for Hiawatha;

Logue went on reading for an hour, entranced by the words. Here was something that really mattered: rhythm—and he had found the door

18

that led him into it.

Even as a young boy, he had been more interested in voices than faces; as the years passed, his interest and fascination in voices grew. In those days, far more emphasis was put on elocution than today: every year in Adelaide Town Hall, four boys who were the best speakers would recite and compete for the elocution prize. Logue, of course, was among the winners.

He left school at sixteen and went to study with Edward Reeves, a Salford-born teacher of elocution who had emigrated with his family to New Zealand as a child before moving to Adelaide in 1878. Reeves taught elocution to his pupils by day and gave 'recitals' to packed audiences in the Victoria Hall or other venues by night. Dickens was one of his specialities. Such recitals were an extraordinary feat not just of diction but of memory: a review in the *Register* of 22 December 1894 described his performance of *A Christmas Carol* in glowing terms: 'For two hours and a quarter, Mr Reeves, without the aid of note, related the fascinating story,' it reported. 'Rounds of applause frequently interrupted the reciter, and as he concluded the carol with Tiny Tim's "God Bless us every one", he was accorded an ovation which testified in a most unmistakable manner to the hearty appreciation of the house.'

In an era before television, radio or the cinema, such 'recitals' were a popular form of entertainment. Their popularity also appears to have reflected a particular interest in speech and elocution throughout the English-speaking world. What could be called the elocution movement had begun to emerge in England in the late eighteenth

19

century as part of a growing emphasis on the importance of public speaking. People were becoming more literate and society gradually more democratic—all of which led to greater attention being paid to the quality of public speakers, whether politicians, lawyers or, indeed, clergymen. The movement took off particularly in America: both Yale and Harvard instituted separate instruction in elocution in the 1830s, and by the second half of the century it was a required subject in many colleges throughout the United States. In schools, particular emphasis was put on reading aloud, which meant special attention was paid to articulation, enunciation and pronunciation. All this went hand in hand with an interest in oratory and rhetoric.

In Australia, the growth of the elocution movement was also informed by a growing divergence between their English and the version of the language spoken back in Britain. For some, the distinctiveness of the Australian accent was a badge of national pride, especially after the six colonies were grouped together into a federation on 1 January 1901, forming the Commonwealth of Australia. For many commentators, though, it was little more than a sign of laziness. 'The habit of talking with the mouth half open all the time is another manifestation of the national "tired feeling",' complained one writer in the *Bulletin*, the Australian weekly, at the turn of the last century.[4] 'Many of the more typical bumpkins never shut their mouths. This is often a symptom of post-nasal adenoids and hypertrophy of the tonsils; the characteristic Australian disease.'

The South Australian accent, with which Logue

grew up, came in for particular criticism as a combination 'polyhybrid of American, Irish brogue, cockney, county, and broken English'. One feature of this was 'tongue-laziness', and an anxiety to 'communicate as much as possible by means of the fewest and easiest sounds'. This laziness was manifest in the clipping of sentences and in the slurring of sounds.

In 1902, aged twenty-two, Logue became Reeves's secretary and assistant teacher, while also studying at the Elder Conservatorium of Music which had been established in 1898 'for the purpose of providing a complete system of instruction in the Art and Science of Music', thanks to a bequest from the wealthy Scottish-born philanthropist Sir Thomas Elder.

Like his teacher, Logue started giving recitals; he also became involved in amateur dramatics. An event on the evening of Wednesday 19 March 1902 at the YWCA in Adelaide allowed him to show off his prowess in both. 'The hall was filled, and the audience was very appreciative,' reported the local newspaper, the *Advertiser* the next day. 'Mr. Logue looks young, but he possesses a clear, powerful voice and a graceful stage presence. He evidenced in his selections considerable dramatic talent—scarcely mature at present, however—and an artistic appreciation of characters he impersonated and of stories he was telling.' The newspaper's critic said Logue had been successful in all the poems and excerpts he had tried, although he was at his best in W. E. Aytoun's 'Edinburgh After Flodden'.

Logue's pride at such reviews was tempered by tragedy: on 17 November that year his father died after a long and painful battle with cirrhosis of the liver at the age of just forty-seven. The following day an obituary of George Logue was published in the *Advertiser* and his funeral was attended by a large number of mourners.

Now twenty-three, Logue was feeling confident enough to set up on his own in Adelaide as an elocution teacher. 'Lionel Logue begs to announce that he has commenced the practice of his profession, and will be in attendance at his rooms, No. 43, Grenfell Buildings, Grenfell Street, on and after April 27. Prospectus on Application,' read a notice published three days earlier in the *Advertiser*. At the same time he was continuing his recitals and even set up the Lionel Logue Dramatic and Comedy Company.

On 11 August 1904 the *Advertiser* published a particularly effusive review of an 'elocutionary recital' that Logue had given at the Lyric Club the evening before, under the headline, 'Next to being born an Englishman, I would be what I am—a "common colonial".' Logue, the reviewer noted, was the 'happy possessor of a singularly musical voice, a refined intonation, and a graceful mastery of gesture, in which there is no suspicion of redundancy'. It concluded: 'Mr. Logue has nothing to fear from his competitors, and his recital was characterised by dramatic expression, purity of enunciation, and a keen appreciation of humour which won him the enthusiastic approval of the audience.'

Then came one of the first of several upheavals in Logue's life. Despite his growing reputation in Adelaide, he decided to up sticks and move more than 2,000 kilometres westwards to work with an

22

electrical engineering firm involved in installing the first electricity supply at the gold mines in Kalgoorlie, Western Australia. The town had grown fast since the discovery of rich alluvial gold deposits in the early 1890s had set off a gold rush. By 1903 Kalgoorlie boasted a population of 30,000, along with ninety-three hotels and eight breweries. The day of the individual prospector was over, however, and large-scale deep underground mining had begun to predominate.

Logue did not stay long, but after completing his contract he had saved up enough money to relax for a few months while he planned the next stage in his life. Not surprisingly, he decided to continue on westwards to the more civilized surroundings of Perth, the state capital. Western Australia had been traditionally regarded as remote and unimportant by those in the east, but that had been changed by the discovery of gold in Kalgoorlie, and Western Australia became a force to be reckoned with especially in the Federation debates prior to 1901.

Installed in Perth, Logue set up another elocution school and also founded the city's public speaking club in 1908. The previous year he had met Myrtle Gruenert, a clerk, who at twenty-two was five years his junior, and who shared his passion for amateur dramatics. An imposing young woman several inches taller than Lionel, she was of German stock: her grandfather, Oskar Gruenert, had come from Saxony in eastern Germany. Her father, Francis, an accountant, was proud of his Germanic roots and was secretary of the Verein Germania club in Western Australia. Francis had been unwell for some time and in

23

August 1905 he had died suddenly aged just forty-eight, leaving behind his wife, Myrtle, forty-seven, Myrtle, then twenty, and her brother, Rupert.

Lionel and Myrtle were married on 20 March 1907 at St George's Cathedral by the Dean of Perth; the event was apparently sufficiently important to warrant a write-up in the next day's edition of the *West Australian*. The bride, as the newspaper reported, was beautiful in a wedding dress of white chiffon glacé silk. A white tulle veil, embroidered at the corners with floral sprays in white silk, was arranged coronetwise on her hair. After the ceremony, there was a reception at the Alexandra Tea Rooms in Hay Street, where Myrtle's mother, dressed in a frock of deep blue chiffon voile, received the guests. The pair spent their honeymoon in Margaret River south of Perth, visiting the caves which had a few years earlier become a major tourist attraction.

The newlyweds went to live at 9, Emerald Hill Terrace. When their first child, Laurie Paris Logue, was born on 7 October 1908, they moved to Collin Street. Myrtle, with whom Logue was to spend the next four decades, was a formidable and energetic character. 'My wife is a most athletic woman,' he told a newspaper interviewer several years later. 'She fences, boxes, swims, and golfs, is a good actress and a fine wife.' She was, he once declared, his 'spur to greater things'.

*　　　*　　　*

It appears to have been Myrtle's idea, two years later, that the two of them should set off for six months on an ambitious round-the-world tour,

24

eastwards through Australia, on across the Pacific to Canada and the United States and then, after crossing America, back home via Britain and Europe. The trip was to be paid for partly from money lent them by Lionel's uncle, Paris Nesbit, a colourful lawyer turned politician. Little Laurie, whose second birthday they had only just celebrated, was to be left behind in the care of Myrtle's mother, Myra.

The inspiration was, in part, a simple desire to see the world. But Logue was also keen to widen his professional experience. By now he had become a well-known figure in Perth through his recitals and the many plays he had directed or appeared in. He was also building up his private practice, working with politicians and other prominent local people to improve their voice production—even though, when asked by a reporter to name some of his patients, he was the soul of discretion: 'Every public speaker likes his hearer to imagine his oratory is an unpremeditated gift of nature, and not the result of prolonged and patient study,' he said, by way of explanation.

America, in particular, was home to many of the leading names in the field of elocution and oratory from whom Logue was keen to learn. Both he and Myrtle also apparently thought that if they liked what they saw on their travels they might settle abroad, sending for their son and Myrtle's mother to join them. The many long letters that Myrtle (and, to a lesser extent, Logue) wrote home were to provide a vivid picture of their voyage.

They set off from home on Christmas Day, 1910, sailing eastwards around Australia, via Adelaide, Melbourne and Sydney to Brisbane, with stops of

25

several days in each. Sydney Harbour, according to Myrtle, was 'wonderful—superb—no language can fit it'. She was less impressed by Brisbane, which she found 'a fearful place—behind the times, unhealthy looking, and hot as Hades'. During the various stops, they had ample opportunity to visit friends and relatives; Lionel—or 'Liney' as Myrtle called him in her letters—impressed the other passengers with his skills at cricket, golf and hockey, and, ever the raconteur, drew on his prowess at public speaking to entertain the passengers and crew with his stories.

Not surprisingly, they were soon missing little Laurie and justifying to themselves the decision to leave him behind. 'I don't let myself think too much of my little son or else I should weep,' Myrtle wrote in one of her first letters to her mother. 'He was so sweet as I left, "Don't cry mummy"—"Don't let him forget me mother dear" . . . The six months will soon pass and we will come back, with wonderful experience and a new outlook on life broadened wonderfully.'

The next leg of their journey across the Pacific proved more traumatic; Logue spent the first eight days of their voyage from Brisbane sick in his bunk and not touching any food at all. It was not just the waves: the drinking water they had taken on in Brisbane was bad and many of the passengers were sick. Logue was convinced he had lead poisoning. 'He is the worst sailor possible, poor old dear—I don't know what would happen to him if he were alone,' wrote Myrtle. 'He has fallen away to a shadow.'

Things looked up after they reached Vancouver and dry land on 7 February. From there they

continued by train through Min[...]
Paul to Chicago, where they too[...]
YMCA overlooking Lake Michiga[...]
a week. The city, wrote Myrtle, w[...]
be one of the wickedest in the worl[...]
to what they had expected, they l[...]
intended to stay only a week or two, [...]
remained for over a month.

Life in a big American city was a fascinating
cultural experience. Myrtle was especially
impressed by the drugstores, where you could buy
anything from patent medicines to cigars, by the
cafes and by the sheer number of automobiles.
However, the lack of manners of the local women,
who 'stare, put their elbows on the table, butter
their bread in the air with their elbows on the
table, pick their chicken bones and use toothpicks
at every conceivable opportunity', was not
appreciated.

The Logues were the toast of the town. Thanks
to friends of friends, some of whom they had met
on the ship, they were invited to dinners at smart
homes and in fancy restaurants and managed to
attend some prestigious functions. They also took
in a number of plays and shows. Lionel was witty
and good company; as Australians, he and Myrtle
must also have been something of a novelty for the
locals. It was not all play, though. By day they went
to Northwestern University, where they attended
classes and lectures given by Robert Cumnock, a
professor of elocution who had founded the
university's School of Oratory, and whom Myrtle
pronounced 'simply charming'. Logue also gave
recitations and talks to students about life in
Australia.

was on via Niagara Falls to New York which amazed them with its sheer size. 'I got an underground railway yesterday and rode nearly an hour, and when I got out, I was still in New York,' Myrtle wrote in amazement.[5] They were also struck by the sheer number of foreigners in the city, many of whom struggled to speak even the most basic English. Broadway, with its miles of 'electric light advertising', dazzled them with its brilliance, and Logue took his wife to her first grand opera. They climbed the Statue of Liberty and enjoyed the amusements of Coney Island. Here, too, the various introductions they had brought from home ensured they were quickly introduced into local society—and treated to some very expensive evenings out on the town. These provided a stark contrast to the harshness of New York life: 'New York is indeed a city of atrocities and lawlessness,' Myrtle wrote to her mother. 'The papers read like Penny dreadfuls, we are never without a revolver, a beauty which Lionel bought on arrival.'

As he had in Chicago, Logue sought out experts in his field, among them Grenville Kleiser, a Canadian-born elocutionist, who wrote a number of inspirational books and self-improvement guides on oratory and elocution. Logue also addressed the local public speaking club and gave talks at the YMCA. During a side trip to Boston, he met Leland Todd Powers, a leading elocutionist who had established the School of the Spoken Word, giving an address to students there and also at the prestigious Emerson School of Oratory.

Intriguingly, during his time on the East Coast Logue also met the future President Woodrow

28

Wilson, who was then head of Princeton University. 'An American of the finest type,' Logue declared in an interview with the Perth *Sunday Times* about his journey when he got back.[6] 'He has keen piercing eyes that seem to look you through and through. A man of great intellect and character, but thoroughly genial and unassuming. Many people think he will be the next President of the United States.' An avid collector of autographs, he treasured a letter written by Wilson in his neat and classical scholarly writing.

It was time to move on. On 3 May Lionel and Myrtle boarded the *Teutonic*, of the White Star line—the company that the following year was to launch the ill-fated *Titanic*—bound for London. Their time in America had been one long adventure. 'We have had a lovely time in America and it is a delightful place to live—but a very bad place to bring up children,' Logue wrote to his mother-in-law. 'The Americans are a wonderful and strange people—it is a country of graft, dishonesty and prostitutes . . . And yet it is one of the most fascinating countries in the world.'

*   *   *

The Logues docked in Liverpool on 11 May and took the four-hour train journey down to London. The English countryside, proclaimed Myrtle in a letter to her mother, was a 'wonderland, picturesque to an extreme, green fields all divided off into lots of these beautiful hawthorn hedges, and the canals with the barges being towed along by an old horse and man on the tow path'. But her first impressions of the capital of the Empire (after dinner and a walk around Piccadilly and Trafalgar Square) were not especially positive; it looked 'provincial' compared with New York.

London quickly grew on them, however, and Myrtle was soon enthusing about what they saw. They did the obvious sights such as the British Museum, the Tower of London, Madame Tussaud's and Hampton Court and, of course, Buckingham Palace—to which Logue, in future years, was to become such a frequent visitor. Myrtle was not impressed by its exterior: 'It's a dirty, ugly grey old place, hideous beyond description, and in front of the gates is the beautiful new memorial to Victoria unveiled a month ago,' she wrote. 'This beautiful piece of work throws into relief the bare monstrosity of Buckingham Palace.'

They made plenty of visits to theatres where they saw, among others, the great Charles Hawtrey, whom they loved, and the Australian-born Marie Lohr, whom they did not: like all English girls, she was too thin and had reached fame far too quickly for her own good, thought Myrtle. She and Logue also ate out a lot, although they were disappointed by the fact that all the restaurants in London closed much earlier than in New York.

They travelled to Oxford, too, where friends of friends invited them for Eights Week, the annual competition in which the colleges' rowers battle it out on the river. They spent the mornings visiting the various colleges and were delighted by the sight of the hundreds of gaily decorated punts from which the men in white flannels and girls in pretty dresses watched the rowers. A friend also took them punting, and they lay back in the cushions as he propelled them along the river under low branches, pointing out all the sights. They left Oxford with the greatest reluctance, after what Logue described in a letter to his mother-in-law as 'six days in paradise'.

One of the highpoints of their visit to Britain was on 22 June when they were among the crowds who turned out on the streets of London for the coronation of King George V, the 'sailor king' who had succeeded his father, Edward VII, in May the previous year. London was a seething mass of humanity and its streets decorated with so much bunting and so many electric lights that it looked to Myrtle like fairyland. People had begun staking out the best vantage points the evening before, sleeping on the pavement, and everyone had to be in their place by six o'clock the following morning. A friend of Logue's named Kaufmann, whom he had met on the *Teutonic*, managed to get him a reporter's pass allowing access right up to the doors of Westminster Abbey.

Armed with the pass, Logue and Kaufmann strolled down at 9.30 and were permitted by the police to pass through to a position just a few hundred yards from Buckingham Palace from which they enjoyed a magnificent view of the King and Queen in their golden carriage. 'It was a very enthusiastic crowd, but the English are all afraid to make a noise,' he wrote to his mother-in-law.

The next day was the royal progress into London proper, and Logue and Myrtle had seats in the Admiralty stand, just outside the new Admiralty Arch. Although they had to wait from 7.15 a.m. until 1.30, the time flew by and they 'behaved like

31

kids when the King and Queen came by in their beautiful state carriage with the eight famous cream horses, each with its postillion and leader'. The Logues also found time to visit Edith Nesbit, author of *The Railway Children*, and a distant cousin of theirs, at her beautiful home in the Kent countryside. It was a trip that Myrtle in particular found enchanting.

They had originally intended to travel on to Europe but now there was a problem: Logue had invested a large chunk of savings in shares in the Bullfinch Golden Valley Syndicate, which had created huge excitement on the Perth Stock Exchange the previous December after claiming to have struck gold in a new mine near Kalgoorlie. The company's predictions proved hopelessly exaggerated, however, and the share price collapsed a few months later, taking most of the couple's savings with it. They cabled Uncle Paris to send some more money, but appreciated the need to economize and went instead to stay with relatives in Birmingham for a few days.

On 6 July they set off for home from Liverpool aboard the White Star Line's SS *Suevic*, a liner designed especially for the Australian run, and later that month the couple arrived back without mishap at King George Sound, Albany, Western Australia. 'Had enough of travelling for a time?' Logue was asked in the same Perth *Sunday Times* interview about his travels in which he had mentioned his meeting with Woodrow Wilson. 'That I have,' he replied. 'Australia is the finest country of the world.'

*   *   *

Back home, Logue was able to draw on his experiences in Britain. When a special coronation programme called *Royal England* was staged in the New Theatre Royal in Perth that August, Logue was chosen to provide the commentary to accompany a show of 'animated pictures specially cinematographed by C. Spencer from privileged positions along the route'.

Logue could scarcely have imagined that one day he would be consulted by the King's son on his speech defects, yet this (and other such performances) were turning him into a notable figure on Perth's social scene. In December 1911 his recently established school of acting, which included many well-known local amateurs, gave their first performance: on the evening of Saturday the 16th they appeared in his production of *One Summer's Day*, a comedy by the English playwright Henry Esmond. Two days later an entirely different cast appeared in a production of *Our Boys*, the proceeds of which were to go to a local nursing charity.

Myrtle, meanwhile, was also beginning to make an impact: in April 1912 the *West Australian* reported she was opening a 'school of physical culture (Swedish) and fencing for women and girls in the Wesley gymnasium', a lofty and well-ventilated hall at the back of Queen's Hall. Myrtle, the article claimed, had 'recently returned from abroad, where she had the advantage of studying the most up-to-date methods in force both in England and America'.

The following month, Logue's troupe was back at His Majesty's Theatre with a production for

33

charity of Hubert Davies's drawing room comedy, *Mrs Gorringe's Necklace*. The beneficiary this time was the Parkerville Waifs' Home. 'Mr. Logue and his pupils are heartily to be congratulated,' declared the *West Australian*. 'There was nothing mechanical about it, no dependence placed upon mere recitative, and the whole thing was a frank and genial appeal to ordinary human nature.' Myrtle, too, joined him on stage: her performance as Mrs Jardine was a 'very artistic bit of work in voice, act, and general manner', the newspaper found.[7]

Logue's own elocutionary recitals, meanwhile, were drawing large and enthusiastic audiences. 'The announcement of a recital by Mr Lionel Logue was sufficient to comfortably fill St George's Hall last night, and those who attended were amply repaid for venturing out on a showery evening,' read one review in August 1914 which described him as 'a master of the subtle art of elocution in all its branches'.

Logue appears to have gone down particularly well with women in the audience—as was noticed by a local newspaper reporter when Logue went back to Kalgoorlie to serve as 'elocutionary adjudicator' at a Welsh-style Eisteddfod, which, according to the account, sounded somewhat reminiscent of a modern-day television talent show. 'Mr Lionel Logue,' the reporter noted, 'is a very good-looking young man and a number of goldfield girls were not slow to appreciate it. Two of them followed up the competitions every evening and spent most of the time gazing soulfully in the direction of the judge's cabinet. It might be interesting for those young ladies to know that Mr Logue has a charming wife and two beautiful children.'[8]

Logue was also enjoying plaudits for his work with his elocution students. In September 1913, at a dinner in the Rose Tea Rooms in Perth's Hay Street (organized by the Public Speaking Club, which Logue had founded five years earlier) several of his pupils 'testified to their appreciation of that gentleman's abilities and to the success of his tuition,' according to one contemporary account. To the amusement of the twenty or so present, one speaker wondered whether Logue might turn his considerable talents to making the large number of politicians and others who posed as public speakers stop talking nonsense and switch to common sense instead. Logue replied in suitably humorous tone, describing the proper use of the mother tongue as 'the first evidence of civilization and refinement'.

However comfortable their life in Perth, Lionel and Myrtle's eyes had been opened by their world tour and they seem to have been slowly coming around to the idea of trying to make a new life abroad, perhaps in London. Any immediate prospect of a move had been dashed by the birth of their second son, Valentine Darte, on 1 November 1913. Then on 28 June 1914 the assassination of Archduke Franz Ferdinand of Austria in faraway Sarajevo forced them to put their plans on hold indefinitely.

*   *   *

For Australia, as for the mother country, the First World War was to prove hugely costly in terms of

35

death and casualties. Out of a population of fewer than five million, 416,809 men enlisted, of whom more than 60,000 were killed and 156,000 wounded, gassed or taken prisoner.

As in Britain, the outbreak of war was greeted with enthusiasm—and although proposals to introduce conscription were twice rejected in a plebiscite, a large number of young Australian men volunteered to fight. Most of those accepted in August 1914 were sent first not to Europe but to Egypt, to meet the threat posed by the Ottoman Empire to British interests in the Middle East and the Suez Canal. The first major campaign in which the joint Australian and New Zealand Army Corps (ANZAC) force was involved was at Gallipoli.

The Australians landed at what became known as ANZAC Cove on 25 April 1915, establishing a tenuous foothold on the steep slopes above the beach. An Allied attack followed by a Turkish counterattack both ended in failure, and the conflict soon settled down into a stalemate that lasted for the remainder of the year. According to figures compiled by the Australian Department of Veterans' Affairs, a total of 8,709 Australians were killed and 19,441 wounded. Gallipoli had a huge psychological effect on the country, denting Australians' confidence in the superiority of the British Empire. The Anzacs quickly acquired hero status—and their heroism was recognized in Anzac Day, which has been commemorated since on 25 April.

Logue was already aged thirty-four and had two sons, but nevertheless volunteered for military service. He was rejected on medical grounds: after he left school, he had fallen heavily while playing football and smashed his knee, which ended any serious sporting activities—or chance of serving in the army. 'I joined a rifle club, but was obliged to give it up as I couldn't march,' he said in a newspaper interview which appeared during the war years. 'I am afraid as a soldier I should lay up for a few weeks after the first long march, and would only be an unnecessary expense to my country.'

Although spared the horrors of Gallipoli, Logue nevertheless set out to do his bit for the war effort. He put his energies into organizing recitals, concerts and various amateur dramatic performances in Perth in aid of the Red Cross Fund, French Comfort Fund, the Belgian Relief Fund and other charities. The programmes were often a curious mixture of the deadly serious and the comic. During one performance by the Fremantle Quartette Party in July 1915, Logue began with what the reviewer described as a 'graphically descriptive recital of "The Hell Gates of Soissons", which deals dramatically with the glorious martyrdom of twelve men of the Royal Engineers in checking the German advance to Paris in September last'. Later he had his audience roaring with laughter at several 'delightfully humorous trifles'. The reviews, as on this occasion, were invariably glowing and the houses full.

Logue had so far concentrated on elocution and drama, but he attempted to apply some of the knowledge of the voice that it had given him to help servicemen suffering speech disorders as a result of shell shock and gas attacks. He scored success with some—including those who had been told by hospitals that there was nothing that could be done for them. Logue's achievements were documented in some detail in an article that appeared in the *West Australian* in July 1919, under the dramatic headline 'The Dumb Speak'.

His first success appears to have been with Jack O'Dwyer, a former soldier from West Leederville, in the Perth suburbs. Earlier that year, Logue had been sitting on a train next to a soldier and watched, intrigued, as he leant forward to speak to two companions in a whisper. 'Mr Logue thought the matter over, and just before he got to Fremantle he gave the soldier his card and asked him to call on him,' the newspaper reported. O'Dwyer, it emerged, had been gassed at Ypres in August 1917 but had been told in London that he would never speak again. At Tidworth hospital on Salisbury Plain suggestive and hypnotic treatment was tried but failed. And so, on 10 March 1919, the unfortunate man had gone to see Logue.

Logue was convinced he could help. So far as he could tell, the gas had affected the throat, the roof of the mouth and the tonsils, but not the vocal cords—in which case there was hope. At this stage, though, it was only a theory. He had to put it into practice. After a week, Logue managed to get a vibration in O'Dwyer's vocal cords and his patient was able to produce a clear and distinct 'ah'. Logue continued, trying to show him how to form sounds, much in the same way as a parent would teach a child how to speak for the first time. Less than two months later, O'Dwyer was discharged, quite cured.

Logue described the treatment (which he made clear to the newspaper that he'd provided without charge) as 'patient tuition in voice production combined with fostering the patient's confidence in the result'—the same mixture of the physical and psychological that was to prove a feature of his future work with the King. As such, it was in sharp contrast to rather more brutal methods, including electric shock therapy that had been tried on patients in Britain—apparently to no avail.

Encouraged by his treatment of O'Dwyer, Logue went on to repeat his success with five other former soldiers—among them a G. P. Till, who had been gassed while fighting with Australian forces at Villers-Bretonneux on the Somme. When he came to see Logue on 23 April that year, Till's vocal cords weren't vibrating and what voice he could muster had a range of just two feet. Logue discharged him on 17 May after he appeared to have made a full recovery. 'In fact, I could not stop talking for about three weeks,' Till told the newspaper. 'My friends said to me, "Are you never going to stop talking?" and I replied, "I've got a lot of lost time to make up."'

CHAPTER THREE

Passage to England

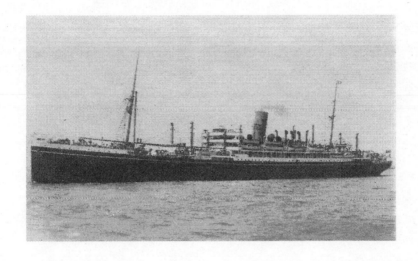

The *Hobsons Bay*, which carried the
Logue family to England

On 19 January 1924 Lionel and Myrtle set off for England aboard the *Hobsons Bay*, a twin-masted single-funnel ship of the Commonwealth and Dominion Line. They travelled third class. With them were their three children, Laurie, now aged fifteen, Valentine, ten and a third son, Antony Lionel (usually known in the family as Boy), born on 10 November 1920. The 13,837-ton ship, which had 680 passengers and 160 crew, had made its maiden voyage from London to Brisbane less than three years earlier. After forty-one days at sea, they steamed into the port of Southampton on 29 February.

It was only by chance—and another of the spontaneous decisions that shaped his life—that Logue, by then employed as an instructor in elocution at the Perth Technical School, had found himself aboard the *Hobsons Bay*. He and a doctor friend had planned to take their families away for a holiday together. The Logue family's bags were packed and their car ready to go when the telephone rang: it was the doctor.

'Sorry, but I cannot go with you,' he said, according to an account later published by John Gordon, a journalist and friend of Logue's.[9] 'A friend has fallen ill. I have to stay with him.'

'Well, that holiday is over,' Logue told his wife.

'But you need a holiday,' she replied. 'Why don't you go out East by yourself?'

'No,' he replied. 'I went East last year.'

'Then why not Colombo?'

'Well,' Logue replied, hesitantly. 'If I went to Colombo I would probably want to go to England.'

'England? Why not!' exclaimed Myrtle.

Rapidly warming to the idea, Myrtle had her husband call a friend who was head of a shipping agency. When Logue asked about the possibility of getting two cabins on a ship to Britain, his friend laughed.

'Don't be silly,' the friend replied. 'This is Wembley year. There isn't a cabin free in any ship, and not likely to be.'

The friend did not need to explain what he meant by Wembley. That April, George V and the Prince of Wales were due to open the British Empire Exhibition, one of the greatest shows on earth, in Wembley in north-west London. The exhibition was the largest of its sort ever staged and intended to showcase an empire at its height that was now home to 458 million people (a quarter of the world's population) and covered a quarter of the total land area of the world. The exhibition's declared aim was 'to stimulate trade, strengthen bonds that bind Mother Country to her Sister States and Daughters, to bring into closer contact the one with each other, to enable all who owe allegiance to the British flag to meet on common ground and learn to know each other'.

Three giant buildings—Palaces of Industry, Engineering and Arts—were constructed; so, too, was the Empire Stadium, with its distinctive twin towers, which as Wembley Stadium became the heart of English football until it was demolished in 2002. Some twenty-seven million people in total visited—many of them from the far corners of the Empire, including Australia.

With all these people heading for Britain, the Logues' prospects of realizing their dream seemed slim, but half an hour later the phone rang again: it was the shipping agent, who seemed excited.

'You are the luckiest man,' he told Logue. 'Two cabin bookings have just been cancelled. You can have them. The ship sails in ten days.'

'I'll tell you in half an hour,' Logue replied.

'It's this minute or never.'

Myrtle nodded and Logue didn't hesitate. 'Right, we take them,' he said.

The journey, which lasted almost six weeks, gave them plenty of time to get to know the passengers and crew. They made a particular friend of the master, a Scotsman named O. J. Kydd, who eight years later was to invite Logue to join him on his holiday at his home near Aberdeen, and showed him Holyrood Castle, Glencoe, the Pass of Killiecrankie and dozens of other places that he had read about as a boy.

It is not clear if Logue and Myrtle were planning to emigrate or merely to have another look at the country they had left a decade earlier. The local press reported Logue wanted to gain more professional experience in Britain, especially in the field of speech defects, and that they would return after twelve months. It was arranged that another elocution teacher, Bessie Durlacher, would take his pupils while he was away. Yet rather than place their furniture in storage, they auctioned it all two days before they left. In any case, there were few ties to keep them in Australia. Both their fathers had long since died; in 1921 Lionel's mother, Lavinia, also passed away; Myrtle's mother, Myra, followed in August 1923.

*   *   *

45

The Britain in which the family landed was a country in turmoil. The First World War had caused an enormous upheaval and putting the country back onto a peacetime footing proved a huge challenge, too. David Lloyd George vowed to turn Britain into a Land Fit for Heroes, but jobs had to be found for the returning soldiers, while the women who had taken their places in the factories had to be coaxed into returning to the home. Optimism quickly faded as the immediate post-war boom turned to bust in 1921, public spending was slashed and the jobless total surged. The war had plunged Britain deeply into debt.

Even the imperial triumphalism symbolized by the events at Wembley was illusory: Britain was finding it difficult to shoulder the economic burdens of defending its empire, which had acquired another 1.8 million square miles of territory and 13 million more subjects thanks to the Treaty of Versailles, in which Lloyd George and the leaders of the other victorious Allied powers carved up the world.

The political landscape was changing, too. Stanley Baldwin, who became Conservative prime minister in May 1923, failed to win a majority in a snap election that December, opening the way for Britain's first Labour government. And so, in January 1924, Ramsay MacDonald, the illegitimate son of a Scottish farm labourer and a housemaid, was asked by George V to form a minority administration, with the support of the Liberals. The King was impressed by MacDonald. 'He wishes to do the right thing,' he noted in his diary. 'Today 23 years ago dear Grandmama died.

I wonder what she would have thought of a Labour Government!'

The government did not last long: Labour was defeated in the election that October, paving the way for the return of Baldwin and the Conservatives, who were to dominate British politics over the next two decades, through the General Strike of 1926, the Depression of the 1930s and, eventually, the Second World War.

Such dark days lay ahead; Logue had more pressing problems. He and Myrtle may have originally intended to come on vacation, but they soon decided to stay longer. But how could he support his family? He started to look around for jobs, but it wasn't easy. He had brought with him savings of £2,000—worth many times more than it is today but still not sufficient to keep a family of five for very long.

The enormity of what he had let himself and his family in for must have begun suddenly to dawn on him. He knew no one and had carried only one introduction: to Gordon, a Dundee-born journalist ten years his junior, who in 1922 had become chief sub-editor of the *Daily Express* (and was to go on, from 1928 until 1952, to become a highly successful editor of its sister paper, the *Sunday Express*). They were to remain on close terms for the rest of Logue's life.

Logue settled his family in modest lodgings in Maida Vale in west London and went around local schools offering his services to help deal with children's speech defects. The work he got brought him some money but he knew that, given how small his savings were, it was not going to be enough for him to raise his family. And so he took

47

what was to prove a momentous decision that reflected the supreme confidence he had in his talents: he rented a flat in Bolton Gardens, South Kensington, and leased a consulting room in 146 Harley Street, placing himself in the heart of Britain's medical establishment.

Most of the buildings in the street dated back to the late eighteenth century, but it was only decades later that the name of Harley Street became synonymous with medicine. One of the first medical men to set up shop there was John St John Long, a notorious quack, who arrived in the 1830s—and was subsequently convicted of manslaughter after one of his treatments that involved wounding a young lady patient in the back went horribly wrong. Others followed, attracted not just by the proximity of well-to-do clients in surrounding streets but also ease of access to King's Cross, St Pancras and Euston railway stations, which brought in patients from elsewhere in the country. By 1873, thirty-six doctors had addresses there; by 1900, the street's medical population had swelled to 157 and ten years later to 214.

Harley Street, in short, was already well on the way to becoming a brand rather than just an address. Location within the street was everything, though. Generally speaking, the lower the number and further south towards Cavendish Square, the more prestigious the address. Logue's building was right up towards its northern end, close to the junction with the busy Marylebone Road that runs east to west across London.

Yet Harley Street was still Harley Street. Quite what the street's other celebrated dwellers made of this rough-hewn Australian in their midst has not been recorded. By the time he arrived, the quacks of old had given way to modern, properly qualified doctors. Logue, by contrast, had no formal medical training at all. But none of his neighbours would have known how to advise people with speech impediments or to understand the distress this caused them.

Setting up a practice was one thing: there was then the more difficult matter of actually acquiring some patients. Logue quickly began to make friends among London's Australian community. Described by his journalist friend Gordon as 'bubbling with vitality and personality', he was the kind of person whom people remembered. And so, gradually, he began to carve out a career for himself, treating a mixture of patients, most of them sent to him by other Australians living in London. He charged hefty fees to the rich, with which he subsidized treatment for the poor. But it was still a struggle: 'I am still battling my way up, it takes time, labour and money in London,' he wrote in a letter to Myrtle's brother, Rupert, in June 1926. 'I must have a good holiday soon or I will be going under.' Always on the lookout for ways of supplementing his income, he had taken a job as a special constable when the country was paralysed by the General Strike the previous month, earning six shillings a day.

Speech therapy—and the treatment of stammering, in particular—was still in its relative infancy. 'Those were pioneer days for speech, and in far off Australia little was known of Curatum speech work and consequently for many years all one could do was to experiment,' Logue recalled

49

years later. 'The mistakes one made in those days would fill a book.'

People appear to have suffered from speech impediments almost since man first started to speak. The book of Isaiah, believed to have been written in the eighth century BC, contains three references to stammering.[10] The ancient Egyptians even had a hieroglyph for it. In ancient Greece, both Herodotus and Hippocrates mentioned stammering, although it was Aristotle who came up with the most informative account of early Greek knowledge of speech defects: in his *Problemata*, he described several forms of speech defects, one of which, *ischnophonos*, has been translated as stammering. He also noted that stammerers tended to suffer more when they were nervous—and less when they were drunk.

The most famous stammerer of the ancient world was Demosthenes. As related by Plutarch in his *Parallel Lives*, he would speak with pebbles in his mouth, practise in front of a large mirror or recite verses while running up and down a hill as a way of fighting his speech impediment. These exercises were said to have been prescribed by Satyrus, a Greek actor, whose assistance he sought. The Roman emperor Claudius, who reigned from AD 41 to 54, also had a stammer, although there is no record of his having attempted to treat it.

Interest grew in speech defects in the nineteenth century, thanks in part to medical progress. By the middle of the century, physiological research was being conducted into sound and how we produced it, as well as into hearing. Much remained still to be discovered: it was not until the middle of the twentieth century that phonation (the articulation of speech sounds) was fully understood. The growing emphasis in the period on elocution also inevitably tended to focus interest on the unfortunate minority for whom producing even a simple sentence was a terrifying ordeal.

One of the first people to write on stammering in modern times was Johann K. Amman, a Swiss physician who lived at the end of the seventeenth century and beginning of the eighteenth, and referred to the affliction as 'hesitantia'.[11] Although his treatment was primarily directed to control of the tongue, Amman considered stammering a 'bad habit'. Writers who followed tended to consider it an acquired characteristic that was largely the result of fear.

As knowledge of human anatomy grew, so more physiological explanations began to be sought that concentrated on body structures involved in the processes of articulation, phonation and respiration. Stuttering was explained as a disturbance in one or the other area of function. Attention tended to be focused on the tongue: for some experts, the problem was that it was too weak; others, by contrast, thought it over energized.

At its most harmless, this pinning of the blame on the tongue led to the prescribing of tongue control exercises and the use of various bizarre devices such as the forked golden plate developed by Marc Itard, a French physician, as a kind of tongue support. Sufferers were also recommended to hold small pieces of cork between their upper and lower teeth. More alarmingly, it also led to a fashion for surgery on the tongue, which was

51

pioneered by Johann Dieffenbach, a German surgeon, in 1840, and imitated widely elsewhere in Continental Europe, Britain and the United States. The precise procedure varied from surgeon to surgeon, although in most cases involved cutting away some of the musculature of the tongue. As well as being ineffective, such medical interventions were also painful and dangerous in an era without effective anaesthesia or antisepsis. Some patients died either directly or as a result of complications.

In his book *Memories of Men and Books*, published in 1908, the Reverend A. J. Church recalled how in the 1840s, as a boy of fourteen, he had been operated on by James Yearsley, MD, of 15 Savile Row, the first medical man to practise as an ear, nose and throat specialist. 'He professed to cure stammering by cutting the tonsils and uvula,' recalled Church. Unconvinced by the efficacy of the surgery, he commented, 'I do not think that the treatment did me any good.'

As time went on, attention began to be focused instead more on the process of breathing and voicing: solutions were sought in breathing exercises and systems of breath control. Writers on the subject, many of them in the German-speaking world, set out to establish which particular sounds were most problematic; they also found that a problem often appeared to lie in making the transition between consonant and vowel. They made other observations, too, such as the fact that sufferers tended to have fewer problems with poetry than with prose, and no trouble at all singing, and that the affliction diminished with age. It was also noted that men suffered disproportionately more than women. Emphasis was put on the use of rhythm as a possible cure.

The emergence of psychology as a separate science, and the development of behaviourism and of the study of heredity, helped lead in the early part of the twentieth century to the development of a new discipline and emerging profession: that of speech and hearing science. On the Continent it tended to remain a speciality within medicine. In Britain, by contrast, doctors tended to seek advice on stammering and other such impediments from those who dealt professionally with voice and speech. The new clinics may have been, in most cases, housed within hospitals and nominally under medical supervision, but the practitioners who staffed them, like Logue, tended to come from schools of speech and drama.

One of the better known names in the field in Britain at this time was H. St John Rumsey, for many years a speech therapist and lecturer at Guy's Hospital in London, who in 1922 wrote a few papers for the medical journal the *Lancet* on speech defects, and outlined his ideas in a book, *No Need to Stammer*, published the following year. Rumsey argued as follows: the two main factors in both speech and song are the production of the vocal tone in the larynx and the moulding of that tone into words by movements of the tongue, lips and jaws. The same organs, of course, are used for both speaking and singing, but while in speech the tendency is to concentrate on the words and to neglect the voice, the opposite is often the case in song. For this reason, he argued, the stammerer can often sing without a problem; he can also often mimic dialects and accents, because in so doing he is being compelled to pay more attention to the vowel sounds.

On one occasion, Rumsey suggested a bizarre cure for stammering: ballroom dancing. It had certainly worked, he claimed, for one twenty-year-old girl who contacted him. 'Now, her stammering is going and she can not only follow but lead a dance,' Rumsey told a reporter.[12] 'Her stammer was due to a lack of rhythm. This, through dancing, she can now feel and see.'

Logue shared Rumsey's emphasis on physical explanations for stammering. As one of his former patients later explained, he believed the problem was attributable to a failure of coordination between the mind and the diaphragm and, once a 'lack of synchronism' set in, it soon became a habit. Logue's cure was based on making patients unlearn all the wrong coordination they had developed and learn to speak all over again. 'But you must remember the key to the whole problem is the diagnosis,' he continued.

Some people fall down on the intake of breath, with others, the diaphragm becomes locked, still others cannot make their minds keep pace with their words. Many people, not ordinarily stammerers, find themselves unable to talk smoothly when highly excited. That is usually an illustration of a third type of defect—the mind running ahead of the wind and articulation. A stoppage occurs until the brain can, so to speak, retrace its steps and untangle the knot.[13]

Logue was to outline his ideas in a slightly

54

different way in a radio talk entitled 'Voices and Brick Walls', which was broadcast on 19 August 1925 from London on 2LO, one of the stations run by the fledgling British Broadcasting Company.[14] The title he chose referred to the three main obstacles he believed stood in the way of good speaking: defective breathing, defective voice production and incorrect pronunciation and enunciation.

Nothing, however, was more distressing than defective speech when it reached the magnitude of a stutter or stammer, he went on.

> I know of nothing which will build so huge a 'brick wall' as this defect; the only consolation being that, with hard work upon the part of the student, it can now be cured in about three months; but the ignorance that is shown under this head is appalling.
>
> People who have these defects can, in most cases, sing quite easily and shout at games without any difficulty; but the ordinary procedure of buying a train ticket or asking to be directed in the street, is untold agony.
>
> Those who had to deal with these cases during and after the war know what a tremendous aid Vocal Therapy was and is—by bringing them the relief of the sung word from the torture of the spoken one.

In his talk Logue then described a curious experiment in which he had managed, by visual means, to lower a voice that was too high pitched. The patient was set in front of a stand containing a number of coloured lights and commanded to make an ordinary vocal sound while he watched the highest light. He was then made to lower the pitch of his ordinary speaking voice while the lights were extinguished one by one. This brought the voice, by a great strain, to a lower pitch. The scale was begun next on a lower tone and the voice broke suddenly and permanently to a lower key.

CHAPTER FOUR

Growing Pains

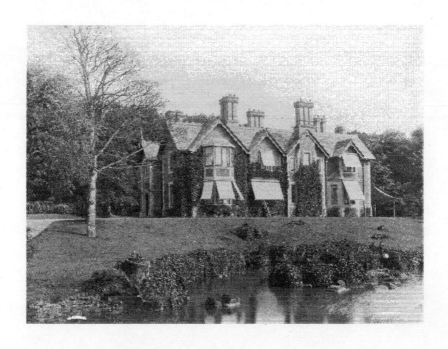

York Cottage, Sandringham.
Birthplace of the future George VI

The future King George VI was born on 14 December 1895, at York Cottage, on the Sandringham estate, on the southern shore of the Wash, the second son of the future George V and a great-grandson of Queen Victoria. Guns boomed in Hyde Park and at the Tower of London. 'A little boy was born weighing nearly 8lb at 3.30 (S.T.) everything most satisfactory, both doing very well,' his father recorded. 'Sent a great number of telegrams, had something to eat. Went to bed at 6.45 very tired.'[15] The S.T. referred not to Summer Time but Sandringham Time, an idiosyncratic tradition adopted by his father Edward VII, a keen huntsman, who set the clocks half an hour early in his own form of daylight saving to allow for more hunting before it got dark.

It was not an auspicious date in the royal calendar: it was on this day in 1861 that Queen Victoria's beloved consort Prince Albert had died at the age of just forty-two. Then on 14 December 1878 her second daughter, Princess Alice, had died at thirty-five. The baby's arrival on what was regarded within the family as a day of mourning and melancholy remembrances was treated with some consternation by the parents.

To everyone's relief, Victoria, by now a venerable old lady of seventy-six, took the birth as a good omen. 'Georgie's first feeling was regret that this dear child should be born on such a sad day,' she wrote in her journal. 'I have a feeling it may be a blessing for the dear little boy, and may be looked upon as a gift from God!' She was also pleased her great-grandson was to be christened

59

Albert, even though he was always to be known to close friends and family as Bertie.

Prince George and his wife Mary—or May, as she was called in the family—already had one son, Edward (or David as he was known), born eighteen months earlier, and there was no secret the couple would have liked a daughter. Others considered the birth of a male 'spare' a good insurance for the succession. After all, George, the second son of the future Edward VII, owed his position as heir to the throne to the sudden death three years earlier of his dissolute elder brother Eddy from influenza that turned into pneumonia, less than a week after his twenty-eighth birthday.

Bertie's early life was spartan and typical of English country house life of the period. The Sandringham estate, which spans 20,000 acres, had been bought by the future Edward VII in 1866 as a shooting retreat. The original house was not grand enough for him and he pulled it down, beginning in 1870 to build a new one that was progressively enlarged over the following two decades in what a local historian described as 'a modified Elizabethan' style. Neither especially ugly, nor especially beautiful, it reminded one royal biographer of a Scottish golf hotel.[16]

York Cottage, given to George and Mary on their marriage in 1893, was a far more modest affair. Situated a few hundred yards from the main house on a grassy mound, it had been built by Edward as overflow accommodation for shooting parties. 'The first thing that strikes a visitor about the house itself is its smallness and ugliness,' wrote Sarah Bradford, the royal biographer.[17] 'Architecturally, it is a higgledy-piggledy building with no merit whatsoever, of small rooms, bow windows, turrets and balconies, built of mixed carstone, a dark reddish-brown stone found on the estate, and pebble-dash, with black-painted half-timbering.' It was also extremely cramped, given that it was home to not just the couple and eventually six children, but also equerries and ladies-in-waiting, private secretaries, four adult pages, a chef, a valet, dressers, ten footmen, three wine butlers, nurses, nursemaids, housemaids and various handymen.

The two boys and Prince Mary, who arrived in 1897, followed by Prince Henry, born in 1900, Prince George in 1902 and Prince John in 1905, spent most of their time in one of two rooms upstairs: the day nursery and the slightly larger night nursery, which looked out over a pond to a park beyond where deer roamed.

Like other English upper-class children of the day, Bertie and his siblings were brought up for the first years of their lives by nurses and a governess who ruled the area beyond the swing door on the first floor to which they were largely confined. Once a day, at tea time, dressed in their best clothes and hair neatly combed, they would be brought downstairs and presented to their parents. The rest of the time they were left entirely in the hands of the nurses, one of whom was later revealed to be something of a sadist. She was jealous of even the little time each day David would spend with his parents and, it was later claimed by the Duke of Windsor in his autobiography, would pinch him hard and twist his arm in the corridor outside the drawing room so he was crying when he was presented to them and

61

quickly taken out again.

At the same time, she largely ignored Bertie, feeding him his afternoon bottle while they were out riding in the C-spring Victoria, a carriage notorious for its bumpy ride. The practice, according to his official biographer John Wheeler-Bennett, was partly to blame for the chronic stomach problems that he was to suffer as a young man. The nurse later had a nervous breakdown.

It was not surprising the children's relationship with their parents was a distant one. Matters were not helped by their father's approach to child rearing. The future King George V had enjoyed what for the era had been a relatively relaxed upbringing, thanks to his father Edward VII, who had been reacting against the strictness with which his parents, Victoria and Albert, had behaved towards him. As a result, whenever she had contact with her grandchildren, the Queen expressed horror at their wayward behaviour.

Far from bringing up his own offspring in an equally liberal way, George did precisely the opposite: the Prince, according to his biographer Kenneth Rose, was 'an affectionate parent, albeit an unbending Victorian'. Thus, although he undoubtedly loved his children, he believed in inculcating a sense of discipline from an early age—influenced in part by strict obedience to authority that had been instilled in him during his and his brother's adolescence in the navy. George wrote a telling letter to his son on his fifth birthday: 'Now that you are five years old I hope you will always try & be obedient & do at once what you are told, as you will find it will come much easier to you the sooner you begin. I always tried to do this when I was your age & found it made me much happier.'[18]

Punishment for transgressions was administered in the library—which, despite its name, was devoid of books, the shelves being filled instead with the impressive stamp collection to which George devoted his leisure time when he was not shooting or sailing. Sometimes the boys would get a verbal dressing down; for serious offences, their father would put them over his knee. The room, not surprisingly, was remembered by the boys largely as a 'place of admonishment and reproof'.

The children's lives changed dramatically following the death of Queen Victoria in January 1901. The Prince of Wales, who now became King Edward VII, took over Buckingham Palace, Windsor Castle and Balmoral, while his son acquired Marlborough House as his London residence, Frogmore House at Windsor and Abergeldie, a small castle on the River Dee near Balmoral. As heir to the throne (and, from that November, Prince of Wales), George began to assume more official duties, some of which took him away from home. That March, he and Mary set off on an eight-month tour of the Empire, leaving their children in the more indulgent hands of Edward and Alexandra. School work was neglected as they followed the round of the Court between London, Sandringham, Balmoral and Osborne; their genial grandfather indulged their boisterousness.

It was also time for the boys to start their education. George had not received much formal schooling himself and did not consider it much of a priority for his own children. David and Bertie were not sent to school but were instead tutored by Henry Hansell, a tall, gaunt tweed-clad bachelor with a large moustache who seemed to have spent more of his time at Oxford on the football or cricket fields than in tutorials or lecture halls. A less than inspiring teacher, he thought the boys would be better off at prep school, like others their age; their mother appears to have agreed. George was having none of it, however, blaming their lack of academic progress on their stupidity. Tellingly, though, he was to relent later with two younger sons, both of whom he sent away to school.

Given the amount of time they spent together—and the distant nature of their parents—it was natural that David and Bertie should become close. It was an unequal relationship: as the oldest child, David both looked after his younger siblings and told them what to do. In his own words, written years later in his autobiography, 'I could always manage Bertie.' As puberty approached, Bertie, like all younger brothers, appears to have begun to resent such management—as Hansell noticed to his concern. 'It is extraordinary how the presence of one acts as a sort of "red rag" to the other,' he reported.[19]

This was more than just usual sibling rivalry. David was not just older, he was also good looking, charming and fun. Both boys were also aware from an early age that he was destined one day to become king. Bertie had been less blessed by fate: he suffered from poor digestion and had to wear splints on his legs for many hours of the day and while he slept, to cure him of the knock-knees from which his father had suffered. He was also

64

left-handed but, in accordance with the practice of the time, was obliged to write and do other things with his right, which can often cause psychological difficulties.

Adding to Bertie's problems—and to some extent a result of them—was the stammer that had already begun to manifest itself when he was aged eight. Indeed, the incidence of stammering has been demonstrated to be higher among those born left-handed. The letter 'k'—as in 'king' and 'queen'—was a particular challenge, something that was to prove a particular problem for someone born into a royal family.

Matters were not helped by the attitude of Bertie's father whose response to his son's struggles was a simple 'get it out'. A particular trial was their grandparents' birthdays, which were marked by a well-established ritual: the children were required to memorize a poem, copy it out on sheets of paper tied together with ribbon, recite the verses in public and then bow and present them to the person whose anniversary was being celebrated. It was bad enough when the poem was in English—later, after they started language lessons, they had to be in French and German, too. Such occasions, to which their grandparents invited guests, were a nightmare for Bertie, according to one of his biographers.

'The experience of standing in front of the glittering company of grown-ups known and unknown, and struggling with the complexities of Goethe's *Der Erlkönig*, painfully conscious of the contrast between his halting delivery and that of his "normal" brother and sister, was a humiliating one which may well have laid the foundation for his horror of public reviews when he was King.'[20]

*   *   *

Like their father before them, the two boys were destined for the Royal Navy. Although for David this was intended as a brief spell before he assumed his duties as Prince of Wales, Bertie was expected to make a career of it. The first stage was the Royal Naval College at Osborne House, Queen Victoria's previous home, on the Isle of Wight. King Edward had refused to take on the house when his mother died and instead gave it to the nation; the main house was used as a convalescent home for officers, while the stable block was turned into a preparatory school for cadets. The experience must have been a strange one for the two boys who had visited 'Gangan'—as Victoria was known—at the house during her final years.

Bertie was thirteen when he was admitted to the college in January 1909; David had arrived two years earlier. It proved a dramatic contrast to Sandringham life for the boys, both socially and intellectually. According to royal tradition, neither of the brothers had been brought up to have contact with other children the same age; by contrast, their counterparts (most of whom had been at preparatory school) would have been used to separation from their parents and to the discipline, harsh conditions, poor food and curious rituals considered an integral part of an upper-class English education.

Then there was the bullying. Far from enjoying preferential treatment from their future subjects as a result of their royal origins, both boys were picked on mercilessly. David, on one occasion, was forced to endure a mock re-enactment of the execution of Charles I in which he was obliged to place his head in a sash window while the other part was brought down violently on top of it. Bertie, nicknamed 'sardine' because of his slight physique, was found by a fellow cadet trussed up in a hammock in a gangway leading from the mess-hall, crying for help. Given the importance placed on team games, the two boys were put at a disadvantage by their lack of experience playing football or cricket.

Bertie's problems were compounded by his dismal academic performance. Osborne was essentially a technical school, concentrating on maths, navigation, science and engineering. Although good at the practical side of engineering and seamanship, he was a disaster at mathematics, typically coming bottom of the class or close to it. Again, his stammer undoubtedly played a role. Although it virtually disappeared when he was with friends, it returned to dramatic effect whenever he was in class. He found the 'f' of fraction difficult to pronounce and, on one occasion, failed to respond when asked what was a half of a half because of his inability to pronounce the initial consonant of 'quarter'—all of which helped to contribute to an unfortunate reputation for stupidity. His father, always better at dealing with his son from afar, seemed to understand. 'Watt [the second master] thinks Bertie is shy in class,' he wrote to Hansell. 'I expect it is his dislike of showing his hesitating speech that prevents him from answering, but he will I hope grow out of it.'[21]

That, however, was going to take several years. In the final examinations, held in December 1910, Bertie came 68th out of 68. 'I am afraid there is no disguising to you the fact that P.A. has gone a mucker,' wrote Watt to Hansell. 'He has been quite off his head, with the excitement of getting home, for the last few days, and unfortunately as these were the days of the examinations he has come quite to grief.'

It was during this time that his beloved grandfather, Edward VII, died. On 7 May Bertie had looked out of his old schoolroom window in Marlborough House to see the Royal Standard flying at half-mast over Buckingham Palace. Two days later, dressed in the uniforms of naval cadets, he and David watched the ceremony as their father was proclaimed King from the balcony of Friary Court, St James's Palace. On the day of their grandfather's funeral, they marched behind his coffin in Windsor from the station to St George's Chapel. The elevation of their father meant David was now first in line to the throne, and Bertie second.

Bertie's dismal academic performance did not prevent him from progressing the following January to the next stage of his education, Dartmouth Royal Naval College, where David was already in his last term. Here again, Bertie faced the inevitable comparisons with his elder brother who was, by any standards, not much of a scholar himself. 'One could wish that he had more of Prince Edward's keenness and appreciation,' wrote Watt.[22]

Matters improved the following year, however,

not least because David left Dartmouth for Magdalen College, Oxford, allowing his younger brother to emerge from his shadow. The curriculum began to be weighted more away from the academic towards the practical aspects of seamanship, to which he was better suited. He was also encouraged by his term officer, Lieutenant Henry Spencer-Cooper, to take up sports that he was better at, such as riding, tennis and cross-country running.

After two years at Dartmouth, he embarked in January 1913 on the next stage of his preparation: a six-month training cruise on the cruiser *Cumberland*. During the voyage through the West Indies and Canada, Bertie experienced the adulation that being a member of the royal family inevitably brought. Such were the number of public appearances that he was required to make that he persuaded a fellow cadet to stand in for him as his 'double' on some minor occasions. He was also confronted for the first time with the need to make speeches, which was to prove such an ordeal for his whole life. A prepared speech he had to read out to open the Kingston Yacht Club in Jamaica proved particularly arduous.

On 15 September 1913, at the age of seventeen, Bertie was commissioned as a junior midshipman on the 19,250-ton battleship HMS *Collingwood*, in the first stage of a naval career, which, like his father before him, he expected to be his life for the next few years. Apparently for security reasons, he was known as Johnson.

There was a major difference between father and son, however. While the future King George V loved both the navy and the sea, his son

69

worshipped the navy as an institution but did not much like the sea itself—indeed he suffered badly with seasickness. He also continued to be plagued by shyness—a fact recorded by several of his fellow officers. One, Lieutenant F. J. Lambert, described the Prince as a 'small, red-faced youth with a stutter', adding 'when he reported his boat to me he gave a sort of stutter and an explosion. I had no idea who he was and very nearly cursed him for spluttering at me.' Another, Sub Lieutenant Hamilton, wrote of his charge: 'Johnson is very well full of young life and gladness, but I can't get a word out of him.[23] Proposing a toast to 'the King' in a Royal Navy wardroom became a torment because of his fear of the 'k' sound.

There were far more serious challenges to come: on 3 August 1914 the United Kingdom declared war on Germany, following an 'unsatisfactory reply' to the British ultimatum that Belgium must be kept neutral. On 29 July the *Collingwood*, together with other members of the Battle Squadrons, had left Portland for Scapa Flow in the Orkneys, off the extreme northern tip of Scotland, with the task of guarding the northern entrance to the North Sea from the Germans.

Bertie went north with his ship but after just three weeks he went down with the first of several medical conditions that were to cast a shadow over his naval career. Suffering violent pains in his stomach and with difficulty breathing, he was diagnosed with appendicitis; on 9 September the offending organ was removed at hospital in Aberdeen.

A semi-invalid at nineteen, while his contemporaries were fighting and dying for his country, Bertie joined the War Staff at the Admiralty. He found the work there dull, however and, after pressing, was allowed back to the *Collingwood* in February the following year. He was on board for only a few months before he began to suffer with his stomach again. He was, it subsequently turned out, suffering from an ulcer, but doctors failed to diagnose it, blaming his problems instead on a 'weakening of the muscular wall of the stomach and a consequent catarrhal condition'. He was prescribed rest, careful diet and a nightly enema, but, not surprisingly, he failed to respond.

Bertie spent much of the rest of the year ashore, initially at Abergeldie, but then at Sandringham, alone with his father, where the two of them became close. During this time Bertie was to learn a lot about what it was to be a king in time of war—an experience that he would be able to draw on when he found himself in the same position two decades later.

In mid-May 1916 he made it back to the *Collingwood*, just in time to take part in the Battle of Jutland at the end of the month. Although again in the sick bay (this time, apparently as the result of eating soused mackerel) on the evening the ship set off, Bertie was well enough to take his place in 'A turret' the following day. The *Collingwood*'s part in the action was not significant, but Bertie was glad to have been involved and, as he recorded, to have been tested by the ordeal of coming under fire.

Much to his relief, his stomach problems appeared to be receding. But then that August they struck again, this time with a vengeance.

Transferred ashore, he was examined by a relay of doctors who finally diagnosed his ulcer. In May 1917, however, he was back at Scapa Flow, this time as an acting lieutenant on the *Malaya*, a larger, faster and more modern battleship than the *Collingwood*. By the end of July, he was ill once more and transferred ashore to a hospital in South Queensferry, near Edinburgh. After eight years of either training or serving in the navy, Bertie realized reluctantly that his career in the service was over. 'Personally, I feel that I am not fit for service at sea, even after I recover from this little attack,' he told his father.[24] That November, after much hesitation, he finally underwent the operation for the ulcer, which went well, however this sustained period of ill health would continue to affect him both physically and psychologically in the years to come.

Bertie was determined not to return to civilian life while the war was going on and in February 1918 was transferred to the Royal Naval Air Service, which two months later was to be merged with the Royal Flying Corps to form the Royal Air Force. He became Officer Commanding Number 4 Squadron of the Boys' Wing at Cranwell, Lincolnshire, where he remained until that August. During the last weeks of the war, he served on the staff of the Independent Air Force at its headquarters in Nancy, and following its disbanding in November, he remained on the Continent as a staff officer with the Royal Air Force.

When peace came, Bertie, like many returning officers, went to university. In October 1919 he went up to Trinity College, Cambridge, where he studied history, economics and civics for a year. It was not immediately clear why he, as the second son, would need such knowledge, but it was to prove more than useful a decade later.

*   *   *

Although Bertie was doing all that was expected of him, his speech impediment (and his embarrassment over it) together with his tendency to shyness, continued to weigh on him. The contrast could not have been greater with his elder brother, who increasingly basked in the adulation of press and public.

Yet all was not quite what it seemed. By the time the two brothers were in their twenties, their relationship with their father began to change. David was already conducting tours of the Empire with great success but those around began to feel that he was enjoying the limelight rather too much for his own—or the country's—good. The King was becoming concerned about his eldest son's almost obsessive love of the modern—which George despised—his dislike of royal protocol and tradition and, above all, the predilection for married women he seemed to have inherited from Edward VII. Father and son began to clash frequently, often over the most minor things such as dress, in which the King took an almost obsessive interest. As the Prince later recorded, whenever his father started to speak to him about duty, the word itself created a barrier between them.

Bertie, by contrast, was gradually becoming his father's favourite. On 4 June 1920, at the age of twenty-four, he was created Duke of York, Earl of Inverness and Baron Killarney. 'I know that you have behaved very well, in a difficult situation for a young man & that you have done what I asked you to,' the King wrote to him. 'I hope you will always look upon me as yr. best friend & always tell me everything & you will always find me ever ready to help you and give you good advice.'[25]

In his capacity as president of the Boys' Welfare Society, which then grew into the Industrial Welfare Society, the Duke, as we will henceforth call him, began to visit coal mines, factories and rail yards, developing an interest in working conditions and acquiring the nickname of the 'industrial Prince'. Starting in July 1921 he also instituted an interesting social experiment: a series of annual summer camps, held initially on a disused aerodrome at New Romney on the Kent coast and later at Southwold Common in Suffolk, which were designed to bring together boys from a wide range of social backgrounds. The last was to take place on the eve of war in 1939.

The Duke rose even further in his father's estimation following his marriage on 26 April 1923 to the society beauty Elizabeth Bowes Lyon. Although his bride had led a life even more sheltered than that of her husband, she was a commoner—albeit a high-born one. The King, who had to give his consent under the Royal Marriage Act of 1772, did not hesitate in so doing. Society had changed, he appeared to have reasoned, making it acceptable for his children to marry commoners—provided they came from among the highest three ranks of the British nobility.

Bertie and Elizabeth had met at a ball in the early summer of 1920. The daughter of the Earl and Countess of Strathmore, Elizabeth was twenty and had just arrived in London society to universal acclaim. A large number of young men were keen to marry her, but she was in no hurry to say yes to any of them—especially the Duke. It was not only that she was averse to becoming a member of the royal family, with all the constraints that this imposed. The Duke also did not seem that much of a catch: although kind, charming and good looking, he was shy and inarticulate, thanks in part to the stutter.

The Duke fell in love with her, but his early attempts to woo her were not successful: part of the problem, as he confided to J. C. C. Davidson, a young Conservative politician, in July 1922, was that he could not propose to a woman, since, as the King's son, he could not place himself in a position in which he might be refused. For that reason, he had instead sent an emissary to Elizabeth to ask on his behalf for her hand in marriage—and the response had been negative.

Davidson had simple advice for him: no high-spirited girl was going to accept a second-hand proposal and so, if the Duke was really as much in love with her as he claimed, then he should propose himself. On 16 January 1923 the newspapers were full of their engagement. Three decades later, after she was widowed, the then Queen Mother wrote to Davidson to 'thank you for the advice you gave the King in 1922'.[26]

Their wedding on 26 April 1923 in Westminster Abbey—being used for the first time for the nuptials of a son of the King—was a joyous occasion. The bride wore a dress of cream chiffon moiré, a long train of silk net and a point de Flandres lace veil, both of which had been lent her by Queen Mary. The Duke was in his Royal Air Force uniform. There were 1,780 places in the Abbey—as the *Morning Post* reported the next day, there was a 'large and brilliant congregation which included many of the leading personages of the nation and Empire'. 'You are indeed a lucky man,' the King wrote to his son. 'I miss you . . . you have always been so sensible and easy to work with (very different to dear David) . . . I am quite certain that Elizabeth will be a splendid partner in your work.'

Yet amid the joy, there was also a reminder that the Duke's marriage was something of a sideshow compared to the occasion when his elder brother would eventually follow suit. In a special supplement, published on the day before the wedding, a writer in *The Times* had expressed satisfaction at the Duke's choice of a bride who was 'so truly British to the core' and had spoken approvingly of his 'pluck and perseverance'. Yet he concluded, as many of the time did, by contrasting Bertie with his 'brilliant elder brother', adding: 'There is but one wedding to which the people look forward with still deeper interest—the wedding which will give a wife to the Heir to the Throne and, in the course of nature, a future Queen of England to the British peoples'. The newspaper and its readers were to be disappointed.

*   *   *

Marriage was a turning point in the Duke's life: he became far happier and more at ease with himself—and with the King. His father's devotion to Elizabeth also helped: although a stickler for punctuality, he would forgive his daughter-in-law her chronic lateness. When she turned up for a meal on one occasion when everyone was already seated, he murmured, 'You are not late, my dear. We must have sat down too early.' The birth of their first daughter, Elizabeth, the future Queen, on 21 April 1926 brought the family even closer together.

They lived initially at White Lodge, in the middle of Richmond Park, a large and rather forbidding property that King George II had built for himself in the 1720s. The couple really wanted to live in London, however, and, after a long search for something suitable within their budget, they moved in 1927 to Number 145 Piccadilly, a stone-built house close to Hyde Park Corner, facing south with a view over Green Park towards Buckingham Palace.

The Duke was continuing with his factory visits and seemed relaxed and happy in such work. More formal occasions—especially speech-making—were a different matter completely, however. The continuing speech defect was weighing on him. The sunny and companionable temperament of his boyhood began to be lost behind a sombre mask and diffident manner. Her husband's impediment and the effect that it had on him were having an effect on the Duchess, too; according to one contemporary account, whenever he rose from the table to respond to a toast, she would grip the edge of the table until her knuckles were white for fear he would stutter and be unable to get a word out.[27] This also further contributed to his nervousness which, in turn, led to outbursts of temper that only his wife was able to still.

The full extent of the Duke's speech problems became painfully obvious for all to see in May 1925, when he was due to succeed his elder brother as president of the Empire Exhibition in Wembley. The occasion was to be marked by a speech that he was due to give on the tenth. The previous year, thousands of people had watched as the slim golden-haired figure of the Prince of Wales had formally asked his father for permission to open the exhibition. The King had spoken briefly in response—and for the first time his words were broadcast to the nation by the then British Broadcasting Company (and later Corporation). 'Everything went off most successfully,' the King noted in his diary.[28]

It was now up to the Duke to follow suit. The speech itself was only short and he practised it feverishly, but his dread of public speaking was making itself felt. Equally terrifying was the fact that he would be speaking in front of his father for the first time. As the great day approached he became increasingly nervous. 'I do hope I shall do it well,' he wrote to the King. 'But I shall be very frightened as you have never heard me speak & the loudspeakers are apt to put one off as well. So I hope you will understand that I am bound to be more nervous than I usually am.'[29]

Matters were not helped by a last-minute rehearsal at Wembley. After he was a few sentences into his speech, the Duke realized no sound was coming out of the loudspeakers and

78

turned to the officials next to him. As he did so, someone threw the appropriate switch and his words, 'The damned things aren't working', boomed around the empty stadium.

The Duke's actual speech, broadcast not just in Britain but around the world, ended in humiliation. Although he managed through sheer determination to struggle his way to the end, his performance was marked by some embarrassing moments when his jaw muscles moved frantically and no sound came out. The King tried to put a positive spin on it: 'Bertie got through his speech all right, but there were some long pauses,' he wrote to the Duke's young brother, Prince George, the following day.[30]

It would be difficult to overestimate the psychological effect that the speech had both on Bertie and his family, and the problem that his dismal performance threw up for the monarchy. Such speeches were meant to be part of the daily routine of the Duke, who was second in line to the throne, yet he had conspicuously failed to rise to the challenge. The consequences both for his own future and that of the monarchy looked serious. As one contemporary biographer put it, 'it was becoming increasingly manifest that very drastic steps would have to be taken if he were not to develop into the shy retiring nervous individual which is the common fate of all those suffering from speech defects'.[31]

*   *   *

By coincidence, Logue was a member of the crowd at Wembley listening to the Duke's speech that

79

day. Inevitably, he took a professional interest in what he heard. 'He's too old for me to manage a complete cure,' he told his son, Laurie, who accompanied him. 'But I could very nearly do it. I am sure of that.' By an equally strange coincidence, he was to get the chance to do precisely that—although it was not to be until a few months later.

There have been different versions of how precisely the Duke was to become Logue's most famous patient, but according to John Gordon of the *Sunday Express*, the chain of events that led to it was set in motion the following year when an Australian who had met Logue afterwards encountered a worried royal equerry.

'I have to go to the United States to see if I can bring over a speech defect expert to look at the Duke of York,' the equerry explained. 'But it's so hopeless. Nine experts here have seen him already. Every possible treatment has been tried. And not one of them has been the least successful.'

The Australian had a solution. 'There's a young Australian just come over,' he said. 'He seems to be good. Why not try him?'

The next day, 17 October 1926, the equerry came to Harley Street to meet Logue. He made a good impression, and the equerry asked if he would be able to meet the Duke and try and do something for him. 'Yes,' said Logue. 'But he must come to me here. That imposes an effort on him which is essential for success. If I see him at home we lose the value of that.'

There is another, more intriguing, version, according to which the role of go-between was played by Evelyn 'Boo' Laye, a glamorous musical comedy star. The Duke had had a crush on her since he first saw her on stage aged nineteen in 1920, and Laye, a lyric soprano, was later to become a friend of both himself and his wife. Five years later, she was appearing at the Adelphi Theatre in the title role of the musical play *Betty in Mayfair* and, after a gruelling schedule of eight performances a week, was beginning to have problems with her singing voice.

According to Michael Thornton, a writer and long-term friend of Laye, the singer sought the advice of Logue, who diagnosed incorrect voice production and prescribed some deep breathing exercises relating to the diaphragm—which quickly relieved her problems. Laye was deeply impressed. And so in summer 1926, when she met the Duchess of York and their conversation turned to the forthcoming trip to Australia and all the speeches that the Duke would have to make there, Laye recommended Logue.

'The Duchess listened with great interest and asked if she would let them have Mr Logue's details,' recalls Thornton. 'The Duchess appeared to consider it a point of great importance that Lionel Logue was an Australian and that she and the Duke were going to Australia.'[32] Shortly afterwards, Laye called Patrick Hodgson, the Duke's private secretary, and gave him Logue's telephone number.

Laye herself continued to consult Logue for many years, especially in 1937 when she was faced with the strenuous role of singing a leading role alongside Richard Tauber, the great Austrian tenor, in the operetta *Paganini*. With Logue's encouragement, she also began to give the future

81

King singing lessons, which were aimed at improving the fluency of his delivery when he spoke.

Whoever was responsible for the initial introduction, the first meeting between the Duke and Logue almost didn't come off. Although his wife was keen he should seek professional advice, Bertie was becoming increasingly frustrated with the failure of the various cures he had been persuaded to try—especially those that assumed his stammering had its root in a nervous condition, which seemed to make matters worse rather than better. The Duchess was determined he give Logue a try, however, and, for her sake if nothing else, he eventually succumbed and agreed to an appointment. Those few minutes were to change his life.

CHAPTER FIVE

Diagnosis

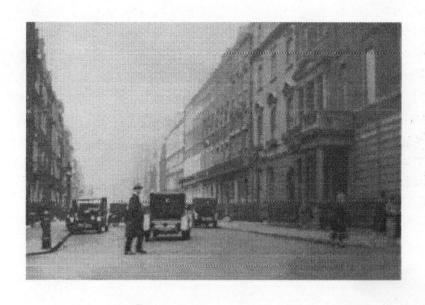

Harley Street in 1926

'Mental: Quite Normal, has an acute nervous tension which has been brought on by the defect . . .' A card, written in a small, spidery hand and headed 'His Royal Highness The Duke of York— Appointment Card', records Logue's first impressions of the Duke of York after he had climbed the two flights of stairs leading to his consulting room in Harley Street at 3 p.m. on 19 October 1926.

'Physical [*sic*]: Well built, with good shoulders but waist line very flabby,' the card entry continued.

Good chest development, top lung breathing good. Has never used diaphragm or lower lung—this has resulted through non control of solar plexus in nervous tension with consequent episodes of bad speech, depression. Contracts teeth & mouth & mechanically closes throat. Gets chin down & closes throat at times. An extraordinary habit of clipping small words (an, in, on) and saying the first syllable of one word and the last in another clipping the centre and very often hesitancy.

During this first meeting, Logue traced his patient's problems to the treatment that he had suffered at the hands of both his father and his tutors, who had appeared to have little sympathy for his speech impediment. The Duke mentioned to him the incident when as a child he had been unable to say the word 'quarter' and his continuing

85

problems with both 'king' and 'queen'.

'I can cure you,' Logue declared at the end of their session, which lasted an hour and a half, 'but it will need a tremendous effort by you. Without that effort, it can't be done.'

Logue identified the Duke's problem, as with many of his patients, to be one of faulty breathing. They agreed on regular consultations. Logue prescribed an hour of concentrated effort every day, made up of breathing exercises of his own invention, gargling regularly with warm water and standing by an open window intoning the vowels one by one, each for fifteen seconds.

Logue insisted, however, that they should meet not at the Duke's home or another of the royal buildings but at either his practice in Harley Street or his small flat in Bolton Gardens. Despite the difference in rank between them, this meeting should be on equal terms—which meant a relaxed relationship rather than the formal kind that a prince would normally have with a commoner.

As Logue later recalled, 'He came into my room a slim, quiet man with tired eyes and all the outward symptoms of a man upon whom a habitual speech defect had begun to set the sign. When he left you could see that there was hope once more in his heart.'

Gradually, progress began to be made—as Logue's case notes, although brief and to the point, reveal:

Oct 30: Diaphragm much firmer, a distinct
    advance.

Nov 16: A good all round improvement much

greater control, diaphragm almost under complete control.

Nov 18: As he progresses the click in the throat becomes very noticeable as other faults are cleared up. Diaphragm is now forcing air through throat muscles.

Nov 19: Never made a mistake during the hour, despite fact very tired.

Nov 20: Lower jaw became pliable.

After the initial interview, the Duke had a total of eighty-two appointments between 20 October 1926 and 22 December 1927, according to a bill eventually drawn up by Logue on 31 March 1928. The initial consultation cost him £24 4s; the other lessons a total £172 4s. Logue charged him a further £21 for 'lessons taken on trip to Australia', giving a grand total of £197 3s—the equivalent of close to £9,000 today.

*   *   *

This 'trip to Australia' was the main reason for the Duke's visits to Harley Street. The following January, he and the Duchess were to embark on a six-month world tour abroad the battle-cruiser *Renown*. The highpoint would be 9 May, when the Duke was to open the new Commonwealth Parliament House in Canberra. It was a highly symbolic occasion. The *Daily Telegraph* claimed the Duke's speech there would be as historic as Queen Victoria's proclamation as Empress of India in

1877. With all eyes—and, more crucially, ears—upon him, Bertie could not risk a repetition of the Wembley fiasco.

The origins of the trip went back just over a quarter of a century to the transformation of the then Australian colonies into states, federated together under one Dominion government. This government, and the parliament to which it was responsible, was initially located in Melbourne, in the State of Victoria. This was only a temporary solution, however; while the people of Victoria would have liked their capital to become the federal one, Sydney, the capital of New South Wales, also wanted the honour.

A decade later, a compromise was finally decided upon: the government acquired an area of nine hundred square miles from the state of New South Wales, which was to be designated federal territory and serve as the site of a new Australian capital, Canberra. Although the First World War caused a hiatus, building work finally began in 1923, and 1927 was chosen as the year for transfer of power to Canberra and the convening of the first session of the federal parliament. Stanley Bruce, the prime minister, asked King George V to send one of his sons to perform the opening ceremony.

The Duke's elder brother, the Prince of Wales, had toured Australia in 1920 to lavish acclaim, and the King felt it was time his younger son carried out an important imperial mission. But he was not entirely convinced that Bertie was up to it—not least because of his stammer. Bruce had his doubts too: he had heard the Duke speak several times during the Imperial Conference of 1926 and had not been impressed. Bertie was equally doubtful about his ability to get through the gruelling programme of speeches that would be required. Embarking on such a long trip would also mean leaving behind his Duchess and their only child, Princess Elizabeth, who had been born the previous April.

Despite such concerns, on 14 July the Governor-General sent a cablegram to the King asking that the Duke and Duchess open parliament; five days later came the official confirmation back from London.

It was against this background that the Duke was to have his first meeting with Logue exactly three months later—and it seems to have provided him with a considerable psychological boost. According to Taylor Darbyshire, an early biographer of the Duke, 'The one great advantage of that first consultation was that it had given the Duke assurance that he could be cured . . . Disillusioned so often before, the change in the outlook caused by the discovery that his trouble was physical and not as he had always feared mental, re-established his confidence and renewed his determination.'[33]

It was one thing to identify the problem but quite another to rectify it. In the seven months leading up to the trip, the Duke would regularly meet Logue for an hour either in Harley Street or at his home in Bolton Gardens. Every spare moment he had outside his official duties was spent on practising and doing exercises that he had been set. If he was out hunting, he would make sure he came back early to put in an hour's work with Logue before dinner. If he was on an official engagement, he would arrange for a break to allow him to fit in his lesson.

'What those seven months imposed upon the Duke in toil and effort has never been adequately understood by the nation,' recalled Logue's friend, the *Sunday Express* journalist John Gordon, years later. All that effort at last began to show results: the Duke began to conquer difficult consonants over which he had previously stumbled. Each breakthrough prompted him to throw himself back into his exercises with still more determination.

On one occasion, a snobbish neighbour sent a curt letter to Logue telling him to instruct his visitor not to park his car outside his house. When the Australian replied that he would tell the Duke to put his car somewhere else, the neighbour's tone changed completely. 'Oh, no, don't. I'll be delighted if the Duke will continue to leave it here.'

A few weeks before he was due to leave on his trip, the Duke faced a test of his speaking abilities. The Pilgrims Society, a dining club with the aim of furthering Anglo-American relations, wanted to hold a farewell dinner for him. Its members, a mix of politicians, bankers, businessmen, diplomats and other influential figures, were used to hearing some of the best speakers in the world. On this occasion Lord Balfour, who had been prime minister more than two decades earlier, was in the chair and some of Britain's most gifted speakers were on the toast list. In short, it would have been a challenge for the best orator, let alone for someone who still struggled to pronounce the letter 'k'.

The Duke decided to confront the challenge head on. He prepared and revised the speech himself and, on the day of the banquet, left the hunting field early to have a final rehearsal with Logue. The Duke's reputation was such that those present hadn't expected much more than a few hesitant words. Instead, they were addressed by a smiling, confident speaker who, although no great orator, spoke with a surprising confidence and conviction. As Darbyshire put it, 'Those who were at that dinner will not easily forget the surprise in store for them.'

Although they had largely tiptoed around the sensitive matter of the Duke's speaking problems, the newspapers also expressed surprise at how well he'd done. 'The Duke of York is rapidly improving as a speaker,' reported the *Evening News* on 27 December. 'His voice is good—unmistakably the family voice. He still sticks too closely to his notes to have much freedom in his manner; but is none the less princely.' Another newspaper added, 'Everybody knows the difficulties under which he speaks. He has practically conquered his impediment of utterance, and as his old private secretary Sir Ronald Waterhouse remarked as the gathering was dispersing, "Wasn't he wonderful! It was the best delivered speech he has ever made."'

The Duke revealed later that he had treated the speech as a real test of the progress he had made under Logue's tutelage and that, by acquitting himself with such success, he had reached a turning point in his career; at last, his handicap seemed to be fading into the past.[34]

The challenges the Duke would face on the tour were of a wholly different scale, however. He would have liked to have his teacher with him but Logue declined, pointing out that self-reliance was an important part of the cure. Pressure was put on Logue to change his mind, but he stood firm, stating it would be a 'psychological error'.

The Duke appears not to have held it against him—an apparent acceptance on his part, too, of the importance of self-reliance. The day before he left, he wrote, 'My dear Logue, I must send you a line to tell you how grateful I am to you for all that you have done in helping me with my speech defect. I really do think you have given me a real good start in the way of getting over it & I am sure if I carry on your exercises and instructions that I shall not go back. I am full of confidence for this trip now anyhow. Again so many thanks.'[35]

The Duke and Duchess sailed from Portsmouth on 6 January 1927. The King and Queen had seen them off at Victoria; there was a particular sadness about their departure—they also had to say farewell to their baby daughter Elizabeth. 'I felt very much leaving on Thursday, and the baby was so sweet playing with the buttons on Bertie's uniform that it quite broke me up,' the Duchess wrote later to the Queen.[36] Frequent letters from home reporting on their daughter's progress went only a little way to comforting them in their absence.

Bertie was also weighed down by the seriousness of the formal responsibilities ahead. Twenty-six years earlier his father, at the time the Duke of Cornwall and York, had inaugurated the federation by opening the first session of the Commonwealth parliament in Melbourne. Now his second son was to follow in his footsteps. 'This is the first time you have sent me on a mission concerning the Empire & I can assure you that I will do my very best to make it the success we all hope for,' he wrote to his father.[37] Determined to give the best performance he could, Bertie embarked on the exercises that Logue had prepared for him. He applied himself to his schedule with considerable energy, even while many of those around him were resting in the tropical heat.

They sailed westwards, stopping at Las Palmas, Jamaica and Panama. In an effusive letter from Panama on 25 January, the Duke described how he had been practising his reading exercises and had made three short speeches—one in Jamaica and two in Panama—all of which had gone well, despite the troublesome heat. 'Ever since I have been here,' the Duke wrote:

I have not been held up for a word in conversation at any time. No matter with whom I have been talking. The reading every day is hard to arrange for any length of time, but I do so at odd moments, especially after exercising when I am out of breath. This has not upset me either.

Your teaching I must say has given me a tremendous amount of confidence and as long as I can keep going and thinking about it all the time for the next few months I am sure you will find that I have not gone back. I don't think about the breathing anymore; that foundation is solid and even a rough sea doesn't shake it when speaking. I try to open my mouth and it certainly feels more open than before. You remember my fear of 'The King'. I give it every evening at dinner on

93

board. This does not worry me anymore.

The letter, as always hand written, was signed 'Yours very sincerely Albert'.[38]

Patrick Hodgson, the Duke's private secretary, was also keen to assure Logue of the progress his pupil was making. 'Just a line—in very hot weather—to let you know that HRH is in great form and the improvement in his speech well maintained,' he wrote in mid-February from onboard ship near Fiji. 'He delivered speeches at Jamaica and Panama very well and though perhaps there is a trifle more hesitancy than when you are near at hand he is full of confidence and altogether much better than I expected he would be in your absence.'[39] Hodgson concluded by promising to write again when the Duke had spoken in public a bit more.

Then it was on westwards to New Zealand. At dawn on 22 February, under pouring rain, they passed the narrow straits into the bay of Waitemata and the port of Auckland. The dreaded speeches began immediately in earnest: on the first morning alone, Bertie had to make three of them. 'The last one in the Town Hall quite a long one, & I can tell you that I was really pleased with the way I made it, as I had perfect confidence in myself & I did not hesitate at all,' Bertie wrote to his mother five days later from Rotorua. 'Logue's teaching is still working well, but of course if I get tired it still worries me.'[40] The ensuing weeks passed in a whirl of dinners, receptions, garden parties, balls and other official functions during which the Duke acquitted himself with distinction. The only potential setback occurred on 12 March when the

Duchess was struck down with tonsillitis and, on the advice of her doctors, went back to Wellington to convalesce at Government House.

The Duke's first thought was to abandon the latter part of his tour of South Island and go back to Wellington with her. Intensely shy by nature, he had come to depend heavily on his wife's support. Such was the enthusiasm with which the Duchess was greeted by the crowds—a foretaste of the welcome that Princess Diana was to receive more than a half century later when she and Prince Charles toured Australia and New Zealand—that Bertie was convinced she was the one the crowds really wanted to see.

The Duke persisted, however, and was pleasantly surprised by the response. Impressed by his self-sacrifice, the crowds gave him an especially warm welcome as he continued his tour alone. When he was reunited with the Duchess on board the *Renown* on 22 March, he could look back with a degree of satisfaction on what he had achieved, even without her by his side.

But the real challenge lay ahead with the Australian leg of their tour, which began four days later when they came ashore in brilliant sunshine in Sydney Harbour. Bertie was apparently undaunted by what awaited him. 'I have ever so much more confidence in myself and don't brood over a speech as in the old days,' he wrote. 'I know what to do now and the knowledge has helped me over and over again.'[41]

The following two months, during which the royal couple travelled from state to state, were every bit as packed with engagements—including, of course, speeches. One of the most emotional the Duke had to make was in Melbourne on 25 April to commemorate Anzac Day, marking the twelfth anniversary of the Gallipoli landings. He carried it off with success.

Then on 9 May came the main event of the trip: the opening of parliament. The Duke had slept badly the night before because of nerves, and he had added to his burden by proposing an extra speech. So many people were expected to attend that he decided to make a brief address to the crowds outside as he opened the great doors of the new Parliament House with a golden key. Dame Nellie Melba sang the national anthem; troops paraded and aeroplanes droned overhead—one of them crashed from four hundred feet about a mile from the reviewing stand, killing the pilot. Although some twenty thousand people were present (and an estimated two million listened at home on the radio) the Duke won the battle with his nerves. It was, wrote General Lord Cavan, his chief of staff, to the King, ' a tremendous success & entirely H.R.H's own idea'.[42]

As he stepped into the small Senate Chamber to make his formal address to members of both houses of parliament, the Duke was hit immediately by the heat, which intensified as the lights were switched on for the photographers and cameramen whose footage was to be distributed by Pathé news to viewers back in Britain. 'So terrific was the light that it raised the temperature of the Senate from 65 to 80 degrees in twenty minutes, in spite of the fact that by special request, one third of it was turned off,' noted Cavan.[43] Yet the Duke pressed on, putting in what all concerned considered an impressive performance.

At the official luncheon the 500 guests joined the Duke in toasting his father in orangeade and lemonade—Canberra was by law completely dry. Such enforced abstinence did little to dampen the Duke's feeling of pride and relief in what he had done; this was reflected in a letter he wrote back to his father in which he paid tribute to the assistance he had received from Logue. 'I was not very nervous when I made the Speech, because the one I made outside went off without a hitch, & I did not hesitate once,' he wrote. 'I was relieved as making speeches still frightens me, though Logue's teaching has really done wonders for me as I now know how to prevent & get over any difficulty. I have so much more confidence in myself now, which I am sure comes from being able to speak properly at last.'[44] The Duke also made sure Logue knew how grateful he was: on the evening of the speech, Hodgson sent his teacher a telegram to his home in Bolton Gardens that read simply: 'Canberra speeches most successful everyone pleased.'[45]

On 23 May the Duke and Duchess finally set off for home, the congratulations still ringing in their ears. 'His Royal Highness has touched people profoundly by his youth, his simplicity and natural bearing,' Sir Tom Bridges, the Governor of South Australia wrote to the King, 'while the Duchess has had a tremendous ovation and leaves us with the responsibility of having a continent in love with her. This visit has done untold good and has certainly put back the clock of disunion and disloyalty twenty-five years as far as this State is concerned.'[46]

The drama was not completely over, however.

Three days after the *Renown* left Sydney Harbour and was making its way through the Indian Ocean, a serious fire broke out in one of the boiler rooms and came close to igniting the ship's entire oil supply. The blaze was put out in the nick of time, but such was its seriousness that at one stage there were plans to abandon ship.

The Duke and Duchess landed in Portsmouth on 27 June, giving the locals a chance to assess Bertie's progress from a speech he made in response to the Mayor's welcome address. Basil Brooke, the Duke's comptroller, who was among those present, wrote to Logue to say how 'really amazed' he had been by what he had heard. 'There was practically no hesitation and I thought it was perfectly wonderful,' he wrote. 'I thought you would like to know this.'[47]

While the Duke's three brothers met him in Portsmouth, the King and Queen greeted him and his wife at Victoria station. During their six months away, the royal couple had travelled thirty thousand miles by sea and several thousand by land. The warmth of the reception they received had demonstrated clearly the high regard in which the monarchy was still held in both Australia and New Zealand, and there was little doubt that, by their presence, they had further strengthened such devotion to Crown and Empire.

Just as importantly, the trip had given the Duke a new confidence in his own abilities. He was acutely conscious of the way his performance had improved his standing in the eyes of the King. Conversations with his father no longer seemed quite as daunting as they once had. 'I mustn't boast and I must touch wood while I write this that

I haven't had a bad day since I have been in Scotland,' he wrote to Logue on 11 September from Balmoral. 'Up here I have been talking a lot with the King & I have had no trouble at all. Also I can make him listen, & I don't have to repeat everything over again.'[48] The Duke said he had also told the King's physician, Lord Dawson of Penn, how he was being treated by Logue and he noticed the difference at once—whereupon the Duke told him he should send all his stammering cases to Logue 'and to no one else !!!'[49]

* * *

At a lunch at the Mansion House where the City welcomed him back, the Duke spoke for half an hour pleasantly, smoothly and with great charm about his experiences on the tour. Logue began to think his patient was not only getting over his problems but even on his way to becoming a really first-class speaker. But however great the progress he had made in Australia, Bertie realized he still had to work on his stammer and on his public speaking. And so, a few days after he returned to London he resumed his regular visits to Harley Street.

In the sessions that followed, the Duke would work on the tongue twisters Logue prescribed for him such as 'Let's go gathering healthy heather with the gay brigade of grand dragoons' and 'She sifted seven thick-stalked thistles through a strong thick sieve'. Despite the huge social gulf between them, theirs turned from a professional relationship to friendship, helped by Logue's frank and straightforward style.

'The outstanding feature of the two years he has spent with me is the enormous capacity for work his Royal Highness possesses,' Logue told Darbyshire, the Duke's biographer. 'When he first began to improve, he visualized what perfect speech was and nothing short of that ideal is going to satisfy him. For two years he has never missed an appointment with me—a record of which he can with justice be proud. He realized that the will to be cured was not enough but that it called for grit, hard work and self-sacrifice, all of which he gave ungrudgingly. Now he is "come to his kingdom" of content and confidence in diction.'

The Duchess, too, was also playing an important (if discreet) role, spurring her husband on. Although much of this was conducted in private, others in his presence occasionally got a glimpse, such as on one occasion when the Duke rose to speak after a lunch and appeared to be struggling more than usual. He was about to give up, when those present saw the Duchess reach out and squeeze his fingers as if to encourage him to continue. He invariably did so.

CHAPTER SIX

Court Dress with Feathers

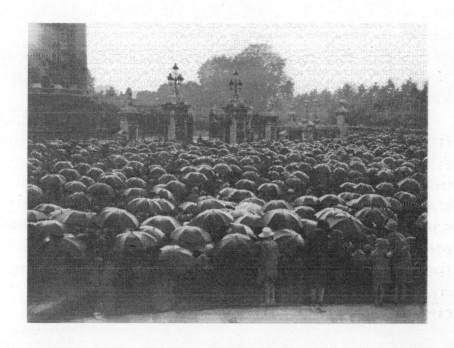

An expectant crowd waiting outside the gates of
Buckingham Palace

The cars were lined up bumper to bumper along almost the entire length of the Mall leading up to Buckingham Palace. It was the evening of 12 June 1928, and a small group of women, dressed up to the nines in feathers and pearls, were about to be presented to King George V and Queen Mary. Most were drawn from the upper echelons of English society; also among them was Myrtle Logue.

This was a rare honour—but one of the perks that now came with Lionel's work. On 20 December 1927 Patrick Hodgson, the Duke's private secretary, had written to say that Myrtle would be presented at one of the next year's Courts by the wife of Leo Amery, the Secretary for the Dominions. On 28 May came the much awaited 'summons' by the Lord Chamberlain to attend the first of two Royal Courts to be held that month at Buckingham Palace.

The card stipulated that ladies were to be dressed in 'court dress *with* feathers and trains'; the gentlemen accompanying them should wear 'full court dress'. Myrtle's attire was suitably grand: a dress of parchment satin over pale pink georgette with diamante shoulder straps and a train of silver tissue, linked with pink tulle, that came right over her left shoulder, fastening on her breast with a diamond buckle, then draped across her back to her right hip with another diamond buckle.

It was just after six o'clock when she and Lionel drove into the Mall, but they barely moved until 8.30 when, one by one, the cars began to edge

103

slowly towards Buckingham Palace, finally arriving at nine. Proceedings were due to start at 9.30. Myrtle's sense of awe at the occasion was mingled with frustration at the long delay and unexpected chaos.

'The wait in the Mall was terrifying,' she wrote in an account of the day later published in an Australian newspaper. 'The "hoi polloi" scrambling on the running board of the car to peer in and see what one's feet looked like! It was too revolting—millions of them—and then, if one looked wearily out into the Mall, one looked straight into the eyes of the young men—and old, too, for that matter—who were cruising up and down in their cars and leering into the carriages. Luckily, Lionel was with me, or I should have died of fright and rage.'

At nine o'clock they were finally allowed inside the Palace and its sumptuous antechamber, where the nodding plumes, tulle veils and jewels made an unforgettable sight. After another wait, this time of about an hour, the Lord Chancellor came for them—the men were taken off to wait in another antechamber and the women stood in queues, their trains tucked over their shoulders. As they entered the throne room, the two equerries whipped the trains off their arms and arranged them on the floor while whispering 'one curtsy to the King and one to the Queen'. As the women's names were boomed out so loudly they almost took fright, they were presented to the King, curtsying without smiling. He responded with a nod, looking seriously at each woman as she passed, before the Queen did the same.

Then, with a fanfare of trumpets, it was all over.

The gentlemen of the bedchamber walked out backwards, carrying their wands of office, followed by the King and Queen, with the pages carrying their trains, bowing right and left as all the women sank to the floor with a curtsy and the men stood to attention, with their heads bowed. Later, feeling flat and tired, Lionel and Myrtle sought out the supper rooms for chicken and champagne. After posing for photographs, they were on their way home. 'I would never have believed it could be such an ordeal,' recalled Myrtle, although she wrote back to Hodgson saying how much she had enjoyed the evening. On 26 July he invited them both to a Garden Party.

At this time the couple bought a little holiday bungalow, named Yolanda, on Thames Ditton Island in the River Thames. It was surrounded by roses and the lawn ran right down to the water's edge. 'Lionel needs a place of rest and peace to go through the spring and summer, and we were getting very tired of taking the children all over the Continent for a month and so missing the loveliest part of the English year, so we decided to stay in England for the summer,' Myrtle explained. 'This place is adorable! We have been down here every week all through the spring and summer. We fish, swim and enjoy boating and just "laze"; and thoroughly enjoy ourselves.'

*   *   *

In the months that followed, the British newspapers increasingly carried articles commenting on the progress that the Duke was making—all of which were collected by Logue and pasted into a large green scrap book that has passed down the family.

Reporting on the Duke's attendance at a fundraising banquet at the Mansion House in London for the Queen's Hospital for Children, the *Standard* noted on 12 June 1928, 'The Duke has vastly improved as a speaker and his hesitation has almost entirely gone. His plea for the children showed real eloquence.' A writer from the *North-Eastern Daily Gazette* came to the same conclusion the following month after a speech by the Duke at another fundraising event for the hospital, this time at the Savoy. 'Taking it all round, I am not sure that his speeches do not equal those made by the Prince of Wales,' the newspaper commented. 'And that is a pretty high standard. The Duke has learnt the speaker's two most valuable lessons—wittiness and brevity. He used rather a good simile at this dinner when he said that he hoped the speakers who followed him would have the effect of the electric plucker he recently saw at an agricultural show—an apparatus which divested a chicken of its external possessions in next to no time.'

The *Evening News* took up the same theme that October. 'The Duke of York grows in fluency as a speaker,' it noted. 'He is markedly more confident than he was two years ago, more confident, indeed, than he was a few months ago. Continued practice tells in public speaking.' The *Daily Sketch* was impressed that the Duke was 'freeing himself more and more from the impediment that formerly interfered with an appreciation of the true gift he possesses for the apt and finished phrase'. Hearing the 'music' in the Duke's voice during a speech at the Stationers' Hall, a somewhat more imaginative writer for the *Yorkshire Evening News* was reminded of other examples of great orators who had overcome hardships. 'I thought of Demosthenes and the story of his victory over hesitant lips; of Mr Churchill and his conquest; of Mr Disraeli whose maiden speech was a humiliation; of Mr Clynes, who in his teens, used to go out into a quarry to practise the art of speaking.'[50]

While newspaper writers noticed the improvement in the Duke's speaking, quite how he had managed to achieve it (and the special role played by Logue) remained a mystery to those who heard him speak, to the wry amusement of his teacher. In another cutting from the period headed 'How well the Duke of York has trained himself to speak', Logue has underlined the phrase 'has trained himself'. In a short report on 28 November 1928, the *Star* attributed the Duke's overcoming of his 'old difficulty in speaking' to the influence of his equerry, Commander Louis Greig, who had become a close friend since they first met almost two decades earlier when Greig was assistant medical officer at Osborne naval college.

Yet it was only going to be a matter of time before the secret got out, given the number of visits the Duke was making to Harley Street and the frequency of Logue's appearances at his side. On 2 October 1928 Logue received a letter at his practice from Kendall Foss, a correspondent in the London office of the United Press Associations of America news agency.

'Dear Sir,' wrote Foss from the agency's office in Temple Ave, EC4.

I understand that you are in possession of the facts concerning the curing of the Duke of York's speech impediment.

Although some miscellaneous information on this subject is current in Fleet Street, I should naturally, like to have the truth before printing this story.

Out of deference for His Royal Highness, I am writing to you for an appointment, hoping that you will be good enough to supply us with the facts for an exclusive story to be published in North America.

Trusting to hear from you favourably, I remain,

Kendall Foss for the United Press.

Logue appears to have rung Hodgson for advice but was told he was 'on holiday, and lost on the Continent'. Foss followed up over the next few days with phone calls both to Harley Street and Bolton Gardens. On 10 October an exasperated Logue wrote back: 'While thanking you for your courteous letter of the 2nd October, it is quite impossible for me to give any information on the subject.'

Undaunted, Foss pressed on with his researches. His story eventually appeared on 1 December 1928 on the front page of the *Pittsburgh Press* and in a number of other US papers. 'The Duke of York is the happiest man in the British Empire,' it began. 'He no longer stutters . . . The secret of the duke's speech defect has been well kept. Since boyhood he has been troubled and for about two years he has been undergoing a cure which has proved

108

successful. Yet the story has never been published in Great Britain.' The account that followed had, Foss wrote, been 'only obtained after the most exhaustive inquiries and investigations. Almost no one in Great Britain seemed able to provide information'.

Foss went on to tell the story of Logue, his techniques and how he had come to work for the Duke. He also noted how in the past, when the royal couple entered a room, the Duchess would step forward and do the talking to save her husband the embarrassment of a stumble. Now, by contrast, he said, 'she hangs back, shyly watching the man of whom she is obviously proud'.

Logue was quoted as merely confirming the Duke was his patient, saying that professional etiquette prevented him from telling more. The Duke's private secretary was equally unwilling to elaborate.

Such reticence did not dampen the journalist's praise for Logue's work. 'Obviously, Logue's analysis of the Duke of York's difficulty was the correct one,' Foss concluded. 'Those who had never heard the Duke speak until recently said they would never dream that he had once suffered agonies of embarrassment over his speech. Much like Demosthenes in ancient Athens, the Duke has mastered a handicap and is making himself into an accomplished orator.'

The floodgates were now open. The following day Gordon's newspaper, the *Sunday Express*, weighed in with its own version—which then went round the world. 'Thousands of people who have heard the Duke of York deliver public speeches recently have commented on the remarkable change in his speech making,' the newspaper wrote. 'The *Sunday Express* is able today to reveal the interesting secret behind it.' The story went on to cover much the same ground as Foss's, noting how what had started as a slight stammer turned into a defect that 'spread its shadow over the whole of the Duke's life', leaving him literally lost for words when he met strangers, with the result that he began avoiding speaking to people.

Despite the closeness of his friendship with Gordon, Logue did not allow himself to be any more forthcoming about his role than he had been with Foss. 'Obviously, I cannot discuss the case of the Duke of York or any other patients of mine,' he told the newspaper. 'I have been asked about this matter many times during the past year by both British and American newspapers and all I can say is that it is very interesting.' The *Sunday Express*'s story was reprinted or followed up by newspapers not only in Britain but also elsewhere in Europe—and especially in Australia, where Logue's contribution was noted with understandable pride.

*   *   *

Perhaps because of the Duke, stammering remained a subject for the press. In September 1929 a debate raged in the pages of *The Times* and other national newspapers over the discovery by scientists that women were far less prone to stammering than men. As 'discoveries' went, it was not a particularly surprising one: people working in the field had long noticed a preponderance of male over female patients. This did not prevent the newspapers devoting many column inches of editorial to it; readers, too, wrote in with their own experiences—even though they differed among themselves as to the cause of the discrepancy between the sexes.

Logue dutifully cut the articles and letters out of the newspapers, pasting them into page after page of his scrap book. Asked by the *Sunday Express* to join the discussion, he came up with his own view—which the edition of 15 September put under the headline, 'Why Women do not stammer. They talk without listening'.

'One reason is that men go out into the world more, and the conditions make them more self-conscious in thinking,' Logue claimed. 'Women will often chatter on to each other without either being concerned in what the other is saying.' As for those women who did stammer, they would do everything to hide their affliction, he added, citing the example of a female patient he had known who travelled every day from the City to her home in Earl's Court, but used to buy a ticket to Hammersmith because she couldn't manage the initial 'k' sound of 'Court'. 'Another would always tender the exact fare on an omnibus, to hide her defect.'

Confirmation of quite how confident the Duke had become about his stammer (and his mastery of it) came the following month with the publication of a book about him by Taylor Darbyshire, a journalist from the Australian Press Association who had accompanied him and his wife on their trip to Australia and New Zealand. The book, running to 287 pages, described itself as a 'an intimate & authoritative life-story of the second son of their majesties the King and Queen by one who has had special facilities, and published with the approval of his Royal Highness'—what we would call today an authorized biography.

The book, which was widely trailed in the newspapers, went into great detail about all aspects of the Duke's life to date. But it was the pages that Darbyshire devoted to his stammer and Logue's work in curing it that most interested the press. Under headlines such as 'How the Duke Won Through', 'Defect in Speech overcome by his pluck' and 'Man who Cured the Duke', they ran details of what one paper called his 'youthful struggle to fit himself to take his place in public life'.

This time, given the Duke's sanction of the book, Logue felt able to talk to the press about his own role—and about the efforts made by his famous patient. 'The real cause of the Duke's impediment was that his diaphragm did not work properly in conjunction with his brain and articulation, and consequently the defect was purely physical,' he said in an interview carried in several newspapers on 26 October. 'As soon as he began to work at the course of voice exercises there was an immediate improvement.

'I have never known a patient so patient and regular,' Logue continued. 'He never missed a single appointment, and he told me he was ready to do anything if he could be cured.' Logue declared that the Duke was, indeed, now cured, 'but he still carries on with physical exercises for the sake of health'. The Duke, he said, was 'the pluckiest and most determined patient I have ever had'.

Word of the Duke's stammer—and of the unconventional Australian who was curing him of it—also spread beyond the British Isles. On 2 December *Time* magazine weighed in with a short article headlined 'Great Britain: C-C-C-Cured'. 'For many years public speaking has been a torture to the stuttering Duke of York,' it said. 'Well known is the fact that in order to avoid saying "K-K-K-King" at moments of state he habitually refers to his father as "His Majesty". Specialists, remembering the Duke's extreme shyness as a child, have for years treated his stuttering psychologically, as caused by nervousness. The treatments were unavailing, His Royal Highness continued to splutter.'

The previous week, it reported, 'Britain rang with joyful news. The Duke's stuttering was so nearly cured that he could say "King" without preliminary cackles. Alone among specialists Dr. Logue had discerned that the ducal impediment was physical, not mental. He had prescribed massage and throat exercises'. Quite where the magazine got the notion that Logue was a doctor was not clear—although he would undoubtedly have been flattered by the title.

The Duke's improvements came despite a worrying scare over his father's health. While attending the Armistice Day ceremony at the Cenotaph in November 1928, the King developed a severe chill, which he neglected and which then turned to acute septicaemia. It became clear he would be incapacitated for some time, and on 2 December six Counsellors of State were appointed to transact public business in the meantime; the Duke was one, as were his elder brother

113

and mother.

Edward was away on a tour of East Africa, and despite warnings of the severity of his father's condition, did not immediately set off for home—to the horror of his aides. Eventually convinced of the seriousness of the situation, he hurried back. During the journey he received a letter from the Duke, which suggested that, despite the gravity of the King's illness, neither brother had lost his sense of humour. 'There is a lovely story going about which emanated from the East End,' wrote the Duke, 'that the reason for your rushing home is that in the event of anything happening to Papa I am going to bag the Throne in your absence!!! Just like the Middle Ages . . .' Edward was clearly so amused by the letter that he kept it and included it in his memoirs.

The King was operated upon and, although his life remained in danger for some time, he began gradually to recover in the new year. It would not be until the following June that he would be strong enough to take part in public ceremonies again. The Duke had been put under strain both by worry about his father and by the extra duties he had to perform, but he took it all in his stride, as he revealed in a letter he sent to Logue on 15 December 1928, thanking him for the book he sent him as a birthday present.

'I don't know whether you sent it with a gentle reminder for me to come and see you more often or not, but I liked your kind thought in sending,' the Duke wrote. 'As you can imagine just lately my mind is full of other things, and as a matter of fact through all this mental strain my speech has *not* been affected one atom. So that is all to the good.'[51]

These birthday books were to become something of a tradition. Regardless of where he was or what he was doing, Logue would send the Duke one or more carefully selected volumes on 14 December for the rest of his life. The Duke, even after he had become King, would respond with a thank-you letter written in his own hand, in which he would inevitably talk about the progress he was making with his speech as well as giving brief insights into other things going on his life. Logue treasured the letters, which found their way into his papers.

CHAPTER SEVEN

The Calm Before the Storm

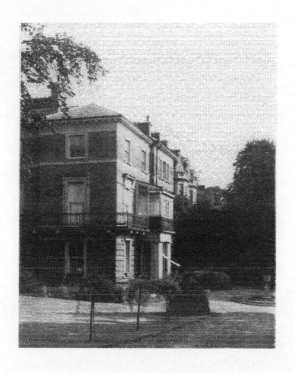

Beechgrove, the Logue family house in Sydenham

The 1930s proved to be the most tumultuous decade of the twentieth century. The Wall Street Crash of October 1929 had brought the Roaring Twenties to a shuddering halt, ushering in the Great Depression, which led to untold economic misery across the world. It also helped the rise of Adolf Hitler, who became German chancellor in January 1933, setting off the chain of events that were to lead to the outbreak of the Second World War six years later.

For the Duke, however, the first six years of the decade, at least, were a time of peace and calm. 'It was almost the last span of untroubled peace that he was to know,' wrote his official biographer, 'and one in which a felicitous balance seemed to have been struck between his arduous duties as a servant of the State and his happy existence as a husband and father.'[52]

Gradually, though, the Duke was being required to play a part in the functioning of the Crown. As well as serving as a Counsellor of State during his father's illness, he had represented him in October 1928 at the funeral in Denmark of Marie Dagmar, the Dowager Empress of Russia, and at the marriage in March the following year of his cousin, Crown Prince Olav of Norway. The same month he was also appointed Lord High Commissioner to the General Assembly of the Church of Scotland. Other duties, and inevitably more speech-making, were to follow.

There were changes, too, on the domestic front: on 21 August 1930, his second daughter, Margaret Rose, was born, and in September the following year the King gave him and the Duchess the Royal Lodge in Windsor Great Park as their country home.

As they grew up, the two princesses were rapidly turning into media stars. Newspapers and magazines on both side of the Atlantic were keen to publish stories and photographs of them—and did so, often with the encouragement of the royal family themselves, who realized their publicity value. Extraordinarily, the third birthday of baby 'Lilibet', as Elizabeth was known in the family, was considered an important enough occasion to earn her a place on the cover of *Time* magazine on 21 April 1929—even though her father, at that stage, was not even heir to the throne.

In the meantime, Logue's personal circumstances were also changing. In 1932 he and Myrtle left Bolton Gardens and moved to the lofty heights of Sydenham Hill, an area largely comprising Victorian villas with generous gardens, offering glorious views towards the city. Their house, 'Beechgrove', at 111 Sydenham Hill, was a sprawling if somewhat shabby three-storey detached property with twenty-five rooms, dating back to the 1860s. It was a few streets away from the Crystal Palace, the giant cast-iron and glass building built to house the Great Exhibition of 1851, which had been erected in Hyde Park but moved to south-east London after the exhibition ended. When the Crystal Palace fell victim to a spectacular blaze in November 1936, drawing crowds a hundred thousand strong, Logue and Myrtle had a ringside seat.

By this time, Laurie was a strapping young man in his late-twenties, almost six feet tall and with an athletic stature he had inherited from his mother. He had gone off to Nottingham to learn the catering business with Messrs Lyons. His brother Valentine was studying medicine at St George's Hospital, which in those days was situated at Hyde Park Corner, while Antony, the youngest, was attending Dulwich College, a mile and a half or so away. The house needed several servants to run, but all the extra space came in useful because the family took in lodgers to boost their income.

To Myrtle's delight, it also had about five acres of garden, including avenues of rhododendrons and a stretch of woodland at the end which, if the rumours were true, had been used to bury the dead during the time of the Great Plague. There was a tennis court, too. As a reminder of home, she succeeded in growing Australian gum and wattle there, although inside the greenhouse rather than outside in the cool London climate.

By this time, Logue's relationship with the Duke was provoking mixed emotions. Like any teacher, he must have felt pride in what he had achieved— yet the more progress his royal pupil made, the less his own services were needed. He nevertheless maintained his contacts with the Duke, writing to him regularly and continuing to send him congratulations and the birthday book. Letters written to him by the Duke, coupled with drafts of those he wrote, were all faithfully glued into his scrapbook.

On 8 March 1929, for example, Logue wrote to the Duke enquiring about how well his speeches were going. 'It is the time when I send a little enquiry to all my patients just to know how they are performing and to ask if speech is quite

121

satisfactory and giving no trouble,' he wrote. 'As I have always treated you just as any other patient I hope you will not mind my enquiry.' Five days later, the Duke wrote back to say that despite the house being full of flu, 'on the few occasions of public speaking all has gone well'.[53]

That September, the Duke wrote to Logue from Glamis Castle, responding to his letter of congratulation on the birth of Princess Margaret Rose. 'We had a long time to wait but everything went off successfully,' he wrote. 'My youngest daughter is going on very well and she has got a good pair of lungs. My wife is wonderfully well, so I have had no worry on that side. My speech has been quite all right and the worry did not effect [sic] it at all.' Then, that December there were the usual royal birthday thanks for 'the little "booook", which is perfect in every way and takes up no room in the pocket'.

The Duke's aides, too, were also taking a great interest in Logue's work with him, as an illuminating handwritten letter from Patrick Hodgson, the Duke's private secretary, sent on 8 May 1930, reveals:

Dear Logue,
    If you can persuade the Duke to try to talk to people more when he goes to functions you will be doing a great service. He is alright at dinner but when people are brought up and introduced to him he has a way of shaking hands, but remaining absolutely mute. I think it is entirely due to shyness, but it makes a bad impression on strangers. I know he funks going up to people and then finding he can't

122

get his words out; but if you can make him believe that it is good for him to make the effort, it would be a real help, because he will have a lot of that sort of thing to do this summer.

Logue's actual meetings with the Duke were becoming rarer, though—despite his attempts, through his letters, to encourage his royal patient to find time for a consultation. Although they met in March 1932, it would be another two years before they would do so again.

'You must be wondering what has become of me,' wrote the Duke on 16 June 1932, from Rest Harrow, Sandwich, Kent, where he and the family had gone to relax for a week. 'You remember me telling you I was feeling unwell and tired in March. I saw a doctor who told me my inside had dropped down and that the lower muscles were weak and so of course I was ill. Now with massage and a belt I am getting better, but it will take time to get perfectly well again. I used to complain to you about my breathing "too low down", as I called it, as those muscles were weak, my diaphragm felt as if there was nothing to hold. Now the breathing is much easier with the aid of the belt, and I talk much better with very little effort.'

The Duke ended his letter by promising to come and see Logue again soon, although he warned he was busy and it might be some time before it was possible. In fact, the visit did not happen that year or the next—largely because of the Duke's growing confidence in his ability to speak in public, which meant such sessions were not necessary.

That September the Duke reflected on the huge

progress he had made since those early consultations with Logue. He continued to have qualms about speaking in public, doing so slowly and deliberately, 'but nothing happens actually during a speech to make me worry any more'. The hesitations were also fewer: Logue advised him to stop pausing between individual words and to pause instead between groups of them.

*   *   *

The Depression was beginning to bite: by the end of 1930 unemployment in Britain had more than doubled from 1 million to 2.5 million—equivalent to a fifth of the insured workforce. Even the royal family felt the need to be seen to make sacrifices (although largely symbolic ones). One of the King's first acts after Ramsay MacDonald, the Labour leader, formed his National Government in August 1931, was to take a £50,000 reduction in the Civil List so long as the emergency lasted. For his part, the Duke gave up hunting and his stable. 'It has come as a great shock to me that with the economy cuts I have had to make, my hunting should have been one of the things I must do without,' he wrote to Ronald Tree, master of the Pytchley Hounds, in Northamptonshire, where he had been hunting for the previous two seasons while renting Naseby House.[54] 'And I must sell my horses too. This is the worst part of it all, and the parting with them will be terrible.'

Those such as Logue who had to work for a living were suffering even more. As everyone tightened their belts, the services he provided would be among the first things on which people

124

would cut back. Although Logue was careful not to be seen to be trading on his royal connection, it must have helped him keep his head above water at such a difficult time. The Duke, ever grateful for what Logue had done for him, made a point of recommending him to his friends.

The coverage Logue received in the *Sunday Express* in December 1928 also appears to have been good for business, as he mentioned in a letter to the Duke the following February. 'Since Xmas I have received over 100 letters from people all over the world asking me to take them as patients,' he wrote. 'Some of the letters are very humorous, but all are pathetic.'[55] Despite this boost, by 1932, the economic downturn was taking its toll, as he wrote to the Duke that January. 'It has been a very hard year for me, as so many people have lost their job.'

Logue, meanwhile, was planning to set up a new clinic, which he told the Duke about in his annual birthday letter in December 1932. Bertie appeared suitably enthusiastic: 'I have been so interested to hear of your new venture with the clinic,' he wrote back on the 22nd. 'I am sure you are right in striking out on your own and feel that so many people know about you now as being the only lasting cure for speech defects. I often tell people about you and give them your address when asked.' The Duke ended his letter with the phrase, 'hoping to see you soon'.

The meeting didn't happen and in May 1934 Logue wrote again, bemoaning the lack of contact, although at the same time praising the Duke on how much his voice was improving. A week later, the Duke responded. 'I am sorry I have not seen you for so long (2 years as you say), but I have very seldom felt that I have needed the help that you can give me,' he wrote. 'This I know is what you want me to feel but at the same time it feels ungrateful of me not to have been to see you.' He went on: 'My belt has done wonders to me in the last two years, and now at last I have had it cut down to a level below the diaphragm, which enables me to breathe without the former support.'[56]

Although busy, the Duke promised to come and see him soon. 'Have you still got your room in Harley Street as I could still run up those stairs, I think,' he wrote.

They did finally get together in 1934—but again it was a one-off meeting.

*   *   *

Logue, meanwhile, was continuing to emerge from the shadows. Following Darbyshire's book, an article appeared about him in the *News Chronicle* on 4 December 1930, in its column 'The Diary of a Man about Town'. Its pseudonymous author, who signed himself Quex, was impressed by the youthfulness of the man who had just celebrated his fifty-third birthday. 'His blue eyes have the flash of youth,' he wrote. 'His hair is crisp and upstanding. He has the schoolboy's complexion, hardly a line on his face, and with the glow that is more English than Australian.'

'Well,' Logue replied. 'I admit I can still run a mile, though I'm not keen on doing it; and you know you can keep young in spirit if you make friends and keep them.'

Reflecting on his career, he noted: 'What really

126

is extraordinary is the number of people who never really hear their own voices. I have tried half a dozen people on the gramophone. They talk into the receiver, and when the voices are reproduced, it is surprising how many are unable to pick out the particular record they have themselves made. No doubt with the average person, the visual memory is more strongly developed than the aural.'

Curiously, Logue claimed his powers of observation were such that, even if he was out of earshot, he could look at a group of people and pick out which one of them was suffering from a speech defect—'Providing they act in a normal way, do not sit still and avoid making their normal gestures.'

Logue outlined his theories in more detail in an article in the *Daily Express* on 22 March 1932. Headlined 'Your Voice May be Your Fortune', it was one of a series of 'Health and Home Talks'. No mention was made of his professional relationship with the Duke, but it is fair to assume readers would have been aware of it. 'The greatest fault of modern speech is the rate at which it is used,' Logue wrote.

There is a mistaken idea that 'hustle' implies achievement, whereas it really means a wrong use of energy and is an enemy of beauty.

The English voice is one of the finest in the world but its effect is often spoiled by wrong production. Only a minimum of people realise what an asset it may be. Was it not Gladstone who said, 'Time and money spent in improving the voice pay a larger interest than any other

127

investment'. This is a strong statement, but I agree with it.

Few people know their own voices because it is difficult to 'hear' oneself. Therefore I advise all who can manage it to hear their own voices reproduced. People are usually surprised when they do this, so seldom do they know how they sound. Speech defects are among the evils of civilisation; they are almost unknown among native races. Nerves account for much of the trouble. The voice is a sure indication, not only of personality, but of physical condition. I have studied voices all my life and can tell a person's physical peculiarities by hearing their speech, even if I am in another room.

Every patient requires slightly different handling and a study of each individual's psychology is necessary. Conditions that will give one man sufficient confidence to overcome a defect will actually set up a similar defect in another.

I once had two brothers as patients. One spoke easily when with his family but could not speak to strangers. The other was fluent with strangers but the reverse with friends or relations. Both were cured but by different methods, although the defects treated were almost identical. Men have almost the monopoly of speech defects. The proportions are one woman to a hundred men.

When a woman has a defect it is usually a bad one, but, she nearly always has success if she decides to overcome it. I think this is due to her power of concentration, which, I always hold, is greater than that of a man.

Stammering is one of the commonest speech defects, and one which can nearly always be cured. In fact, except in rare cases of physical malformation, most speech defects can be overcome provided the will is present in the patient. Without that will to get better, treatment is hopeless. I have had patients to whom I have had to say: 'I can do nothing for you,' [but] given the co-operation of the patient, even extreme cases of aphonia (complete loss of voice) are treatable.

As part of his goal of bringing greater respectability to his profession, Logue also succeeded in setting up the British Society of Speech Therapists in 1935. The Duke was among those whom he told. Logue sent him a copy of the Society's inaugural newsletter. The Duke wrote back, suitably enthusiastic, on 24 July 1935. 'I am so glad to hear you have been able to get your dream in material form at last and do hope it will be a success,' he wrote.

The Society's stated aim was 'to establish the profession of speech therapy on a satisfactory basis in this country and overseas, and to up and maintain suitable standards of professional conduct, consistent with a close relationship with the medical profession'. Many of its members, like Logue, were teachers with experience as private practitioners; some were on the staff of hospitals. Later, the Society was to set up a National Hospital School of Speech Therapy where, after a two-year course in which they studied a range of subjects including phonetics, anatomy, paediatrics, orthodontics and diseases of the ear, nose and throat, students qualified as Medical Auxiliaries (Speech Therapists).

Inevitably, given the sheer number of people with stammers (and the desperation of many to find a cure), the area was an attractive one to quacks keen to cash in. The Society's executive council was especially alarmed in the summer of 1936 by the activities of a certain Ramon H. Wings, a self-styled 'specialist in the German method of the treatment of stammering and stuttering', who placed huge advertisements in Tube stations, on hoardings and in the public press, promising free lectures and advice. Wings's lectures drew audiences of up to a thousand people in search of a quick guaranteed cure for their trouble.

Once the patients had been lured in, they would be given a free personal consultation, at which they would be offered a course of ten lessons for a fee of ten guineas. They would then be divided into groups of twenty to a hundred people, and after a few sessions the best of them would themselves become teachers, and in some cases actually stage big public meetings of their own, producing a kind of snowball effect. After the ten lessons, Wings himself would move on to another city and start the whole process again. All in all, the whole thing was a rather lucrative venture.

The members of the executive were angered by Wings's promises of a quick cure, which they felt aroused unrealistic hopes in patients. Admittedly, such group sessions with a charismatic leader could, through a process of mass suggestion, lead to a marked improvement in 'certain neurotic

130

cases'—during which the glowing testimonials for future advertisements were secured. But such improvements were only temporary. Conditions such as stammering, stuttering, lisping, cleft palate and retarded speech could only be treated over time and on a one-to-one basis. Their concern was clearly not just about their patients; they were equally worried by the effect of such unfair competition on their own members who, as members of the Society, were barred from taking out advertising in any form and obtained their patients on the basis of referrals from the medical profession.

In a letter to the Under-Secretary of State in the Aliens Department, dated 2 October 1936, the Society demanded action against Wings. 'Mr. Wings is making from £5,000–£10,000 a year, and the majority of that comes from exploiting credulous and ignorant people,' they claimed. 'Unless something is done, and done quickly, to stop this unfair competition, and the snowball method of increasing the number of so-called Specialists giving free lectures, followed by courses of treatment, our British Speech Therapists will find themselves left with only their hospital and gratuitous work, and little else. Patients who have once been disillusioned over a reputed cure, generally take years before they will again trust themselves to anyone, in an endeavour to cure their defect.' It is not clear whether any action was taken.

*　　　*　　　*

In December of that year the Duke wrote again to

Logue after he praised a speech he had made. 'On the whole I am very pleased with the continued progress,' the Duke said. 'I take a lot of trouble over practising my speeches, I still have to change words occasionally. I am losing that "sense of fear" gradually, very gradually sometimes. It depends so much on how I am feeling and on what subject I am to speak.'

With the Duke making such progress Logue, now aged fifty-five, may have been reconciled to the fact that their work together was largely over. He would have been wrong. The Duke's life was about to change for ever—and with it Logue's.

Ever since George V's illness in 1928, there had been concerns about his health; a renewal of his bronchial trouble in February 1935 necessitated a period of recuperation at Eastbourne. The King recovered sufficiently to take full part in celebrations of his Silver Jubilee that May, when he appears to have been genuinely surprised at the enthusiastic welcome he was given by the crowds. 'I'd no idea they felt like that about me,' he said, on returning from a drive through the East End of London. 'I am beginning to think they must like me for myself.'[57] When he appeared at Spithead that July to review the Fleet, many onlookers were convinced that he would go on to reign for several more years.

Any improvement was relative, however. The King, who had just celebrated his seventieth birthday, was ailing, and after he returned from Balmoral that autumn, those closest to him noticed a serious deterioration in his health. The death of his younger sister, Princess Victoria, early in the morning of 3 December, came as a

132

tremendous blow and for once his overwhelming sense of public duty faltered—he cancelled the State Opening of Parliament. He went to Sandringham that Christmas for the usual celebrations and made his broadcast to the Empire, but listeners could detect the deterioration in his health.

On the evening of 15 January 1936 the King took to his bedroom at Sandringham, complaining of a cold; he would never again leave the room alive. He became gradually weaker, drifting in and out of consciousness. 'I feel rotten,' he wrote in the last recorded entry in his diary. On the evening of the 20th his doctors, led by Lord Dawson of Penn, issued a bulletin with the words that were to become famous: 'The King's life is moving peacefully towards its close.'

That close came at 11.55 p.m., scarcely an hour and a half later—hastened along by Dawson, who admitted in medical notes (which were made public only half a century later) to have administered a lethal injection of cocaine and morphine. This, it seems, was in part to prevent further suffering for the patient and strain on the family, but also to ensure the death could be announced in the morning edition of *The Times* rather than 'the less appropriate evening journals'. The newspaper, apparently advised to hold its edition by Dawson's wife in London, whom the doctor had tipped off by telephone, duly obliged. 'A Peaceful Ending at Midnight' was its headline the next morning.

The Duke was grief stricken. The consequences for his own life were also dramatic. Although he was carrying out his fair share of royal duties, he had hitherto remained largely in the background. With his elder brother's accession to the throne as Edward VIII, Bertie was elevated to become heir presumptive, which meant he had to take over many of the activities Edward had hitherto carried out. 'All we at 145, Piccadilly knew in the schoolroom was that all of a sudden we saw much less of handsome golden-headed Uncle David,' wrote Marion 'Crawfie' Crawford, the children's nanny. 'There were fewer occasions when he dropped in for a romp with his nieces.'

CHAPTER EIGHT

Edward VIII's 327 Days

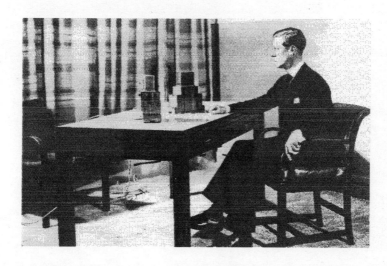

Edward VIII at the beginning of his short reign

No British sovereign ascended the throne with more accumulated goodwill than Edward, the eldest son of George V. Whether because of his courage, his radiant good looks or his avowed concern for the ordinary man (and woman), the new King seemed to embody all that was best about the twentieth century. 'He is gifted with a genuine interest . . . in all sorts and conditions of people, and he is rich in a study that is admirable and endearing in any man and inestimable in a sovereign—the study of mankind,' enthused *The Times* on 22 January 1936. His reign was to last less than year, however, ending in one of the greatest crises the British monarchy has ever endured—obliging his younger brother to take a throne he had not wanted and for which he had not been prepared.

Although noted from an early age for his charm and good looks, Edward had been a shy youth. Then in 1916, at the age of twenty-two, he was introduced by two of his equerries to an experienced prostitute in Amiens who, according to one account, 'brushed aside his extraordinary shyness'.[58] From then on, he seemed to be making up for lost time.

Like his grandfather Edward VII before him, Edward adored London night life. Diana Vreeland, a well-connected fashion columnist, appears to have coined the term the 'The Golden Prince' and declared that all women of her generation were in love with him.[59] Edward showed little interest in the attempts of his strait-laced parents to find him a suitable bride, and instead indulged in a series of affairs, most scandalously one that lasted sixteen years with Freda Dudley Ward, the wife of a Liberal Member of Parliament. After ending the relationship simply by rcfusing her telephone calls, the Prince moved on to Thelma, Lady Furness, the American-born wife of Viscount Furness, the shipping magnate, and twin sister of Gloria Vanderbilt. The couple had a brief affair.

It was at her husband's house, Burrough Court, near Melton Mowbray, either in 1930 or 1931 (depending on whose account you believe) that Thelma introduced the Prince to her close friend, Mrs Wallis Simpson. A fairly attractive, stylishly dressed woman in her mid-thirties, she had been born Bessie Wallis Warfield in 1896 into an old Pennsylvania family that had fallen on hard times—an experience that appeared to have left her with an acquisitive streak. In 1916, aged just twenty, she married Earl Winfield Spencer, an American airman, but he was a drunk and they divorced in 1927. A year later she moved up in the world, marrying Ernest Simpson, an American businessman based in London with connections in smart society.

As the Duke of Windsor was later to recall in his memoirs, their relationship got off to a curious start. Casting around for a bland topic with which to start a conversation, he asked whether, as an American, she suffered from the lack of central heating while visiting Britain. Her reply surprised him. 'I am sorry, Sir,' she said, a mocking look in her eyes, 'but you have disappointed me.'

'In what way?' replied the Prince.

'Every American woman who comes to your

138

country is always asked that same question. I had hoped for something more original from the Prince of Wales.'[60]

The directness of her approach endeared her to Edward, who spent much of his time surrounded by sycophants. Initially they appeared to have been just friends, but this turned to an affair after Thelma went back to America in January 1934 to visit her sister. Then, that summer, the Prince invited Wallis and her husband on a cruise aboard the *Rosaura*, a 700-ton ferry that had just been converted into a luxurious pleasure cruiser by Lord Moyne, a businessman and politician whose family founded the Guinness brewing firm. Ernest had to decline because he had to go on a business trip to America, but Wallis went on her own. It was at this point, she subsequently claimed, that she and the Prince 'crossed the line that marks the indefinable boundary between friendship and love'.[61]

The fact that the Prince of Wales should have a mistress—even a married American one—was not especially problematic, even if the mood of the age was rather different from the time when a previous holder of the title, the future Edward VII, had been pursuing women across London. Provided that she remained a mistress, that is. But the Prince of Wales appeared unwilling to follow his predecessor's acceptance of a distinction between those women who could serve as mistresses and those who had the appropriate background to make them a potential queen. This meant trouble—although it was to take a few months.

After he became King, Edward's popularity grew with his love of all things fashionable and modern.

139

During a visit to the coal mining villages of South Wales, especially hard hit by the Depression, he delighted the crowd by declaring that 'something must be done'. Those around him were less impressed: he dismissed many Palace officials whom he saw as symbols and perpetuators of an old order and alienated many of those who remained by cutting their salaries in the interest of balancing the royal books—yet at the same time spending lavishly on jewels for Wallis from Cartier and Van Cleef & Arpels.

To the exasperation of ministers, Edward was often late for appointments or cancelled them at the last moment. His Red Boxes containing the state papers on which monarchs were meant to work so diligently, were returned late, often apparently unread or stained by the bases of whisky glasses. The Foreign Office took the unprecedented step of screening all the documents they sent to him. Edward was quickly growing tired of what he described as 'the relentless grind of the King's daily life'; George V's warning that, as monarch, his eldest son would 'ruin himself within a year' was beginning to look prescient.

The King was distracted—and the source of his distraction was not difficult to find. Yet he faced a serious impasse: Wallis Simpson was not going to go away; nor would he have allowed her to. In an attempt to square the circle, there was talk of making her Duchess of Edinburgh or of a morganatic marriage—that is one in which none of the husband's titles and privileges pass to the wife or to any children, even though there was no precedent for such a union in Britain. To the alarm of all political parties, there was even a

140

suggestion that Edward might take his fate to the country.[62]

Stanley Baldwin, the Conservative prime minister, and other members of the political establishment considered Mrs Simpson totally unsuitable to be Queen—and feared the heads of the Dominion governments felt the same way. As head of the Church of England, Edward could not be married to a twice-divorced woman with two living husbands. Rumours circulated that she exerted some kind of sexual control over him; there were suggestions she had not just one but two other lovers beside him. Some even said she was a Nazi agent.

As long as Wallis remained married to Ernest, their affair was a potential scandal rather than a political and constitutional crisis. Yet matters were progressing on that front, too. Although there seemed little doubt that it was Wallis's adultery with the King that precipitated her marital break-up, it was customary among gentlemen keen to spare their wives' blushes that they should pose as the guilty party. Ernest had chosen 21 July, the eighth anniversary of his marriage, to be caught *in flagrante* by staff at the swanky Hotel de Paris at Bray on the Thames near Maidenhead with a Miss 'Buttercup' Kennedy. The following month, the King and Mrs Simpson set off on another cruise— this time through the Eastern Mediterranean on board the steam yacht *Nahlin*. Their journey was covered widely in the American and European press, but their British counterparts maintained a self-imposed silence.

So when the case came to court on 27 October at Ipswich Assizes (chosen on the grounds that a

141

hearing in London would attract too much attention from the press), it was Wallis who was divorcing her husband for adultery rather than vice versa. The town had never seen the like.[63] With the King's chauffeur at the wheel, Wallis swept into Ipswich in a Canadian Buick at such speed that a news cameraman's car following at 65 mph was left behind. Security around the courtroom was tight: all newsreel crews had been sent out of town, and two photographers had their cameras smashed with truncheons. Access to the courtroom was also restricted: the mayor, himself an Ipswich magistrate, was admitted only after arguing with his own police officers. All courtroom gallery seats faced by Mrs Simpson as she stood in the witness box were vacant. Tickets were issued only for a few seats to which her back was turned.

Members of staff of the Hotel de Paris then took the stand and described how they had brought morning tea to Mr Simpson and found a woman who was not Mrs Simpson with him in his double bed. After nineteen minutes it was all over and Wallis was granted her *decree nisi*, with costs against her husband. After she left the court, police locked the doors behind her for five minutes to hold the press at bay. Her Buick flashed out of Ipswich as fast as it had arrived and the police swung one of their cars squarely across the road after her, blocking traffic for ten minutes.

Edward and Wallis were not yet free to marry, however. Under the divorce law of the time, the *decree nisi* could not be made absolute for six months—which meant that, formally speaking, she would be under the surveillance of an official known as the King's Proctor until 27 April 1937. If,

142

during that period, she was discovered in compromising circumstances with any man she could be hauled back into court and, if the decision went against her, be forever unable to divorce her husband in an English court. This was only a formality. As *Time* reported, some thirty-six hours after obtaining her decree, Wallis 'was supping gaily in the Palace with the King and a very few friends'. Afterwards, Edward 'squired' her back to her home on Cumberland Terrace.

The clock was now ticking—and the government faced a dilemma. While the American papers offered salacious blow-by-blow accounts of the affair, the British press continued to exercise extraordinary self-restraint. *The Times*, the newspaper of record, did report the divorce but only at the foot of a column of provincial news items on an inside page. American and other foreign newspapers brought into Britain that contained stories about the King and Mrs Simpson's relationship had the relevant columns blacked out or pages removed.

There were limits to how long the cover-up could be maintained, not least because of Britons who travelled abroad and read or heard on the radio about what was happening back home. On 16 November Edward invited Baldwin to Buckingham Palace and told him he intended to marry Mrs Simpson. If he could do so and remain King, then 'well and good', he said—but if the governments of Britannia and its Dominions were opposed, then he was 'prepared to go'.

The King did have some prominent supporters, though, among them Winston Churchill, Britain's future wartime prime minister, who was shouted down by the House of Commons when he spoke out in favour of Edward. 'What crime has the King committed?' Churchill demanded later. 'Have we not sworn allegiance to him? Are we not bound by that oath?' Initially, at least, he also appeared to have thought Edward's relationship with Mrs Simpson would fizzle out, just as his various earlier liaisons had done.[64]

*   *   *

Logue will have watched the unfolding of the dramatic events of December 1936 with as much surprise and shock as King Edward's other subjects. His relations with the Duke of York had also been put on the back burner, although he did receive an invitation to attend a garden party on 22 July at Buckingham Palace.

There were important developments, too, on the Logue domestic front: that September his eldest son Laurie, who was second in command of the ice cream department at Lyons, married Josephine Metcalf from Nottingham. His doctor son Valentine, five years Laurie's junior, was now on the staff at St George's Hospital, where he was awarded the prestigious Brackenbury Prize for surgery. 'I wanted him to follow in my job—but he is set on being a surgeon,' Logue wrote to the Duke.

In the meantime, he had not given up on reviving his royal connection. On 28 October—the day after Wallace Simpson obtained her *decree nisi*—Logue wrote yet again to the Duke suggesting a meeting. 'It was in July 1934 that I last had the honour of speaking with your Royal

144

Highness', he wrote, 'and although I follow all you do and say with the greatest of interest, it is not the same as seeing you personally, and I was wondering if you could spare the time out of your very busy life to come to Harley St—just to see that all the "machinery" is working properly.'[65]

*   *   *

The Duke could be excused for not responding to Logue's proposal: the crisis surrounding his brother's relationship with Mrs Simpson was moving towards a climax and, for the time being at least, he had more pressing matters than his speech impediment.

On 3 December the British press broke their self-imposed silence about the affair. The catalyst was a bizarre one: in a speech to a church conference, Alfred Blunt, the appropriately named Bishop of Bradford, had talked about the King's need for divine grace—which was interpreted, wrongly as it turned out, by a local journalist in the audience as a none-too-veiled reference to the King's affair. When his report was carried by the Press Association, the national news agency, the newspapers saw this as the signal they had all been waiting for: they could report about the monarch's love-life.

Over the previous few months, only a relatively small number of Britons had known what was going on. Now the newspapers quickly made up for lost time, filling their pages with stories of crisis meetings at the Palace, pictures of Mrs Simpson and interviews with men and women in the street asking them their opinion. 'They have much in common,' began a gushing profile of the royal couple in the *Daily Mirror* on 4 December. 'They both love the sea. They both love swimming. They both love golf and gardening. And soon they discovered that each loved the other.'

The Yorks had been in Scotland for the previous days. Alighting from the night train at Euston on the morning of 3 December, they were confronted with newspaper placards with the words 'The King's Marriage'. They were both deeply shocked by what it might mean for them. When the Duke spoke to his brother, he found him 'in a great state of excitement'. The King had apparently not yet decided what to do, saying he would ask the people what they wanted him to do and then go abroad for a while.[66] In the meantime, he sent Wallis away for her own protection. She was receiving poison pen letters and bricks had been thrown through the window of the house she was renting in Regent's Park. There were fears that worse was to come.

The same day the Duke telephoned his brother, who was holed up in Fort Belvedere, his retreat in Windsor Great Park, to make an appointment, but without success. He kept trying over the next few days but the King refused to see him, claiming he had still not made up his mind about his course of action. Despite the huge impact that the decision he made would have on his younger brother's life, Edward did not seek his advice.

Many people spend their careers dreaming of having the top job, but the Duke had no desire to become King. His sense of foreboding was growing. The Duke was 'mute and broken' and 'in an awful state of worry as David won't see him or

146

telephone,' claimed Princess Olga, the wife of Prince Paul of Yugoslavia and sister of the Duchess of Kent.[67] On the evening of Sunday 6 December the Duke rang the Fort to be told his brother was in a conference and would call him back later. The call never came.

Finally, the next day, he made contact: the King invited him to come to the Fort after dinner. 'The awful and ghastly suspense of waiting was over,' the Duke wrote in his account. 'I found him [the King] pacing up & down the room, & he told me his decision that he would go.'[68] When the Duke got home that evening, he found his wife had been struck down with flu. She took to her bed, where she remained for the next few days as the dramatic events unfolded around her. 'Bertie & I are feeling very despairing, and the strain is terrific,' she wrote to her sister May. 'Every day lasts a week & the only hope we have is in the affection & support of our family & friends.'[69]

Events moved swiftly. At a dinner on the eighth attended by several men, including the Duke and the prime minister, the King made it clear he had already made up his mind. According to Baldwin's account, he 'merely walked up and down the room saying, "This is the most wonderful woman in the world."'

The Duke, meanwhile, was in sombre mood. It was a dinner, he wrote, 'that I am never likely to forget'.

At 10 a.m. on 10 December, in the octagonal drawing room of Fort Belvedere, the King signed a brief instrument of abdication in which he pledged to 'renounce the throne for myself and for my descendants'. The document was witnessed by the

147

Duke, who now succeeded him as George VI, as well as their two young brothers, the Dukes of Gloucester and of Kent.

The next evening, after a farewell dinner with his family at the Royal Lodge, the man who was no longer king made a broadcast to the nation from Windsor Castle. He was introduced by Sir John Reith, the director-general of the BBC, as 'His Royal Highness the Prince Edward'. 'I have found it impossible to carry on the heavy burden of responsibility and to discharge the duties of king as I would wish to do without the help and support of the woman I love,' he declared. Edward's reign had lasted just 327 days, the shortest of any British monarch since the disputed reign of Jane Grey nearly four centuries earlier.

After returning to the Royal Lodge to say his familial goodbyes, he left just after midnight and was driven to Portsmouth, where the destroyer HMS *Fury* was waiting to take him across the Channel to exile. As the enormity of what he had done began to dawn on him, he spent the night drinking heavily and pacing up and down the officers' mess in a state of high agitation. The Duke of Windsor, as he would henceforth be known, travelled on from France to Austria where he was to wait until Wallis's divorce was made absolute the following April.

On 12 December, at his Accession Council, the Duke of York, now King George VI, declared his 'adherence to the strict principles of constitutional government and . . . resolve to work before all else for the welfare of the British Commonwealth of Nations'. His voice was low and clear but, inevitably, his words were punctuated by hesitations.

Logue was among those to write his congratulations when he sent his usual birthday greetings two days later. 'May I be permitted to offer my very humble but most heartfelt good wishes on your accession to the throne,' he wrote. 'It is another of my dreams come true and a very pleasant one.' Seeing a chance of reactivating their old ties, he added: 'May I be permitted to write to your Majesty in the New Year and offer my services.'[70]

*   *   *

The newspapers greeted the resolution of the crisis and arrival of the new king with enthusiasm. Bertie may not have had the charm or charisma of his elder brother, but he was solid and reliable. He also had the benefit of a popular and beautiful wife and two young daughters, whose every move had been followed by the press since their birth. 'The whole world worships them today,' declared the *Daily Mirror* in a story about Princess Elizabeth and Margaret, whom it called 'the great little sisters'.

Some foreign observers allowed themselves a more cynical aside. 'Neither King George nor Queen Elizabeth has lived a life in which any event could be called of public interest in the United Kingdom press and this last week was exactly as most of their subjects wished. In effect a Calvin Coolidge entered Buckingham Palace with Shirley Temple for his daughter,' commented *Time*.[71]

Looming over the King was the question of his speech impediment. Thanks to Logue, he had

149

made huge progress since his humiliating appearance at Wembley a decade earlier, but he was not completely cured of his nervousness. For obvious reasons, the tactic adopted was not to draw attention to it, which meant Logue was appalled when Cosmo Lang, the Archbishop of Canterbury, mentioned his stammer in a speech on 13 December, two days after the abdication.

In what shocked many of those listening, Lang, a highly influential figure, had begun his words with an attack on the former King who, he said, had surrendered the high and sacred trust placed in him to a self-admitted 'craving for private happiness'. 'Even more strange and sad it is that he should have sought his happiness in a manner inconsistent with the Christian principles of marriage, and within a social circle whose standards and ways of life are alien to all the best instincts and traditions of his people,' the Archbishop thundered. 'Let those who belong to this circle know that today they stand rebuked by the judgment of the nation which had loved King Edward.'

The directness of the Archbishop's comments promoted an angry response from several people who wrote in to the newspapers—and distressed the Duke of Windsor who listened to this news from the castle in Enzesfeld, Austria, where he was staying with Baron and Baroness Eugen Rothschild.

Ultimately more damaging, however, was what the Archbishop had to say about the new King. 'In manner and speech he is more quiet and reserved than his brother,' he said. 'And here may I add a parenthesis which may not be unhelpful. When his people listen to him they will note an occasional and momentary hesitation in his speech. But he has brought it into full control and to those who hear, it need cause no sort of embarrassment, for it causes none to him who speaks.'

The Archbishop clearly thought his words were for the best. In a speech the following day in the House of Lords, he praised the new King's 'sterling qualities'—his 'straightforwardness, his simplicity, his assiduous devotion to public duty'— which, even though he did not say so directly— were clearly in direct contrast to the brother whom he had succeeded.

Archbishop Lang's comments were picked up by the American press. 'The 300 Privy Councillors were asked by all their intimates one question: "Does he still stutter?"' reported *Time* on 21 December. 'No Privy Councillor could be found willing to be quoted as saying that His Majesty does not still stutter.'

Although the British press refrained from discussing such matters, Lang's comments helped fuel a whispering campaign of gossip against the new King and his fitness to rule. This grew in intensity after he announced in February that he was postponing a Coronation Durbar in India which his brother had planned for the following winter, blaming the postponement on the weight of duties and responsibilities he had faced since his unexpected accession to the throne. For some, though, it was taken as a sign of weakness and frailty; several among the Duke of Windsor's dwindling band of allies suggested Bertie might not be able to survive the ordeal of the coronation, let alone the strains of being King.

151

Back in Australia, Bertie's accession to the throne had led the newspapers to refocus attention on the role of one of their own in helping cure his speech impediment. A rare note of dissent, however, was struck in the letters column of the *Sydney Morning Herald* on 16 December 1936 by one H. L. Hullick, honorary secretary of the Stammerers' Club of New South Wales, who took exception to Logue's diagnosis of the King's speech disorder as physical in nature.

> I have ample authority [Hullick wrote] for stating that no stammer has a physical cause.' This theory was discarded in the 19th century and was at any time but a poor guess without any logical basis. Stammering is an emotional disorder and unless this fact is taken into consideration in giving treatment, the voice condition cannot be relieved.
>
> As a life-long stammerer who has only recently obtained release, I can appreciate better than anyone the struggles his Majesty must have experienced in overcoming his impediment, and this consolidates my deep respect for him. I know nothing of Mr Lionel Logue but have heard of at least four other gentlemen who also claimed to have cured the Duke of York of stammering.

Hullick's letter provoked a spirited response from several other correspondents, including an Esther Moses and Eileen M. Foley of Bondi, whose letter was published on 24 December:

We wish to inform the secretary of the Stammerers' Club of a few facts concerning Mr. Lionel Logue, of Harley Street, formerly of South Australia, and of his undoubted successful treatment of his Majesty, King George VI, then the Duke of York.

During a visit to London in 1935 and 1936, we were the privileged guests of Mr. and Mrs Logue in their private home at Sydenham Hill, and are therefore in the position to prove to your correspondent that without doubt Mr. Logue did cure his Majesty of his stammering, after all other specialists had failed.

In vindication of this statement we have read letters, personally written by his Majesty, to Mr. Logue, in which he gratefully thanked him for the success of his treatment. This was effected just prior to the Royal visit to Australia of the Duke and Duchess of York in May, 1927, and greatly contributed to the success of their tour.

Much credit is given to her Majesty Queen Elizabeth, who during the entire trip, untiringly carried out instructions, personally given her by Mr. Logue. Your correspondent writes that he has heard of at least 'four other gentlemen' who claim to have 'cured the Duke of stammering.' Can he, or any of these four gentlemen, produce similar evidence of the success of their treatment?'

CHAPTER NINE

In the Shadow of the Coronation

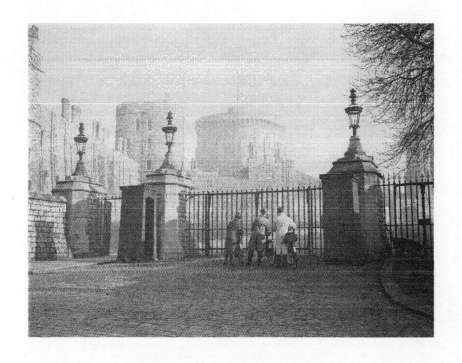

Windsor Castle in 1937

On 15 April 1937 Logue received a call asking him to go and visit the King at Windsor Castle four days later. He was not told the purpose of the visit, but it was not too difficult to guess. 'Hello, Logue, so glad to see you,' said the King, dressed in grey clothes with a blue stripe, coming forwards with a smile as he walked into the room. 'You can be of great help to me.' Logue, ever the professional, was pleased to notice that his former patient's voice had become deeper in tone, just as, all those years ago, he had predicted it would.

The reason for the invitation soon became clear. On 12 May, after five months as King, Bertie was to be crowned in Westminster Abbey. It was to be a massive event, dwarfing in scale George V's jubilee in 1935 or indeed his coronation that Logue himself had attended more than two decades earlier during his round the world trip. Every town had decorations in the streets, while shops in London were competing with one another to produce the most impressive displays of loyalty to the monarch. Huge crowds of people were expected to converge on the capital.

For the King, the main cause for concern was the ceremony itself, particularly the responses he would have to make in the Abbey. Would he be able to speak the words without stumbling over them? Just as daunting was the live broadcast to the Empire he was due to make that evening from Buckingham Palace.

As the occasion approached, the King became increasingly nervous. The Archbishop suggested he try a different voice coach but Dawson, the physician, rejected the idea, saying he had full confidence in Logue. The King agreed. Alexander Hardinge, who had been Edward VIII's private secretary and was now fulfilling the same role for his successor, wondered if it might help to have a glass of whisky or 'some other stimulant' before speaking; this, too, was rejected.

At their first preparatory meeting, teacher and patient went through the text of the speech the King was to deliver in the evening, making considerable alterations. Logue was pleased to find that the King, although a bit stiff about the jaw, was in excellent health and, he recalled, 'most anxious to do best'.

Before he left, Logue remarked how much better the King seemed—to which he replied that he wouldn't have taken on the job twelve years earlier. The conversation also turned to Cosmo Lang and the unfortunate remarks he had made about the King's speech impediment. It was, said Logue, 'a terrible thing that the Archbishop had done'—especially since there was a whole generation growing up who did not think of their monarch having problems with his speech.

'Are you gunning for him, too?' laughed the King. 'You ought to hear what my mother says about him.'[72]

Such concerns began to fade after the King went, together with members of the royal family and Lang, on Friday 23 April to unveil a monument to his father, making his first speech as monarch. Logue, who went along to watch the ceremony, was pleasantly surprised to hear how many people openly expressed astonishment at how well the King spoke. Particular satisfaction

158

came when he overheard one of the onlookers say to his wife, 'Didn't the Archbishop say that man has a speech defect, my dear?' To Logue's amusement, the wife replied, 'You shouldn't believe what you hear, dear, not even from an Archbishop.' The following Monday the King went downriver to Greenwich to open a new hall. He had a wonderful reception and spoke well, although Logue noted he was having trouble with the word 'falling'. Two days later, at Buckingham Palace, there was another speech, this time to acknowledge a gift he was given from Nepal. It was, Logue recalled, 'a nasty speech' and had some particularly awkward words in it.

Nevertheless the main challenge still lay ahead: on 4 May, at 5.45 p.m., Logue met Sir John Reith to check that the microphone was properly installed. It was fitted to a desk to enable the King to broadcast while standing up, as was his preference. He tried it out, speaking some of the words from the text of the planned broadcast speech. He had also been at a rehearsal at the Abbey and had been amused that everyone there seemed to know their job except the bishops.

After a few moments the two princesses came in, saying 'Daddy, Daddy, we heard you'. They had been listening in a nearby room where a loudspeaker had been installed to relay the two men's voices. After staying a few minutes the little girls wished Logue what he described as a 'bashful good night' and, after shaking hands with him, went to bed themselves.

The King continued to practise over the next few days but with mixed results. On the sixth, with the Queen listening, things went badly and he became almost hysterical, although she managed to calm him down. 'He is a good fellow,' Logue wrote of the King, 'and only wants careful handling.' The next day, with Reith and Wood (the BBC sound engineer) in attendance, they recorded a version of the speech. It was too slow and the King was disgusted with it. They tried again, but halfway through he wanted to cough, so they had to make yet another attempt. 'He was quite pleased and departed for his lunch in good patter and with his normal happy grin,' Logue wrote. 'He always speaks well in front of the Queen.'

On the seventh, Reith, who was taking a close interest in the speech, was able to write to Logue that all the gramophone records made that morning were in a sealed box that had been left with a Mr Williams at the Palace. He suggested making a composite record of them, 'which could be more or less perfect as to speech, by taking bits of the first attempt and bits of the third, so that there need be no blemishes anywhere'. This, Reith thought, would not only be handy in case anything went wrong on the twelfth; it could also be used for transmissions of the speech planned for the Empire throughout the night and the next day, and might also be given to HMV as the basis of a gramophone they were planning to sell.

Writing back, Logue insisted the final decision was up to Hardinge, but added, 'A good record is essential, just in case of accidents, loss of voice etc, and the third one with the treatment you suggest, should make an excellent record.'

While the records provided a useful insurance policy of sorts, the King was further encouraged by eulogistic reports in the newspapers the next day of a speech he had made in Westminster Hall. It was, Logue agreed, 'a good job it was not in front of a microphone. It is partly his dislike of the microphone, it must have been engendered when he returned from SA [South Africa] and made his first speech in Wembley Stadium. It was a terrible failure and the scar has remained ever since.'

While there would be no dreaded microphone in the Abbey, the King would have to make his speech into one that evening. Logue was not sure whether it would be better to have a dozen people present or for him to be there alone with the King. 'In an ordinary speech, he is ever nigh perfect, he makes a good speech, and enjoys it but loathes the microphone,' he wrote in his diary.

Logue decided the room on the first floor opposite the King's study was an excellent room for broadcasting, because it looked out onto the main quadrangle and was very quiet. A steward had discovered an old desk in the basement, which had been covered with baize and its sloping lid raised up by two blocks of wood until the top was level. Two gilt microphones and a red light were mounted between them. 'We have tried sitting down to a small table, but he is better on his feet,' Logue wrote. 'He is indeed a gallant fighter, and if a word doesn't quite go right, he looks at me so pathetically and then gets on with the job. There is very little wrong with him, the only big thing is "fear".'

The same day Logue received a call from his friend John Gordon, now already six years into his tenure as editor of the *Sunday Express*. The coronation, and speculation about how well the King would speak his lines, was inevitably reviving

161

the newspapers' interest in his speech impediment —and in the assistance Logue had given him in fighting it. Gordon read him an article about the King which, Logue was pleased to note, did not mention him at all by name. Even after all these years, he was still trying to avoid rather than seek out the limelight.

An hour later, Gordon called him to say that a Mr Miller, who claimed to be a reporter on the *Daily Telegraph*, had sent in an article to the *Sunday Express* about the King that began: 'A black eyed grey haired man, aged 60, an Australian, is in constant attendance on the King and is his greatest friend. They ring each other up every day, etc. etc.'

It was, Logue considered, 'all wrong. Very scurrilous and would do a tremendous lot of harm. John asked if he had my authority to act. I said of course, that it was a damn shame that such a thing should be written. John sent for him and said that the article was quite wrong and could cause a lot of harm. He put the fear of hell into Mr Miller and said that if he sent it to anyone, he would never have another article published. Mr Miller left the article with John and said that it would not happen again. John rang me up and told me the good news. Thank Heavens.'

On the morning of Monday the tenth, with two days to go before the coronation, Logue went to the Palace. The tension was clearly getting to the King, whose eyes looked very tired. 'He said he was not sleeping well and his people didn't even know what was the matter,' recorded Logue. 'Think he is very nervy.'

That evening, at eight o'clock, there was another twist. Logue received a telephone call saying he

162

was being recognized in the Coronation Honours List for his services to the King. He didn't believe it at first and rang Gordon, who confirmed its veracity. Later he and his family went over to Gordon's house, drank champagne and celebrated. Clearly thrilled, Logue ended his diary that day, 'Everything Splendid. "M.V.O."—Member of the Victorian Order.'

When Logue saw the King the following afternoon, he thanked him for the great honour. The King grinned and said, 'Not at all. You have helped me. I am going to reward those who help me.' He then took the order out of his drawer, showed it to Logue and said 'wear this tomorrow'. The Queen laughed and congratulated Logue.

While he was there, Logue and the King listened through the recording they had made of his speech. It was good enough to broadcast, but Logue hoped it wouldn't be necessary to use it. 'H.M. improves every day, getting good control of his nerves and his voice is getting some wonderful tones into it,' he noted in his diary. 'Hope he does not get too emotional tomorrow. H.M. offered up a prayer tonight. He is such a good chap—and I do want him to be a marvellous King.'

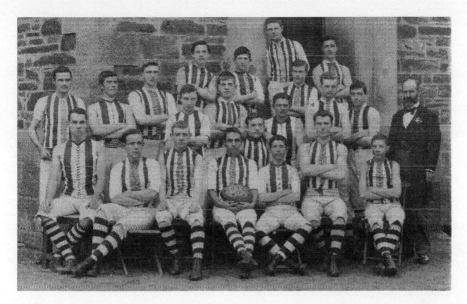

Prince Alfred College inter-college football team 1896
Lionel stands beneath the
teammate leaning against
the doorway

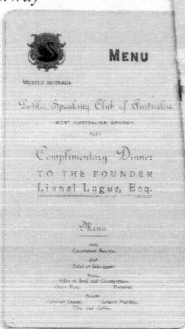

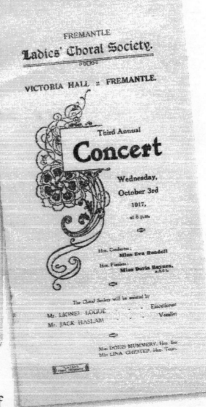

Menu for a dinner given in
honour of Lionel and a
concert programme for one of
the many recitals he gave

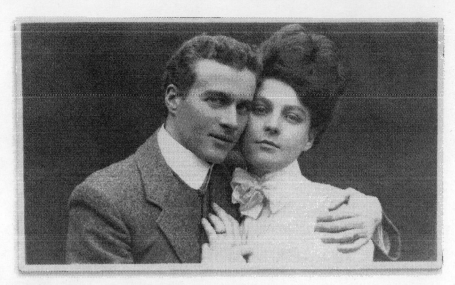

Lionel Logue and Myrtle Gruenert on their engagement, 1906

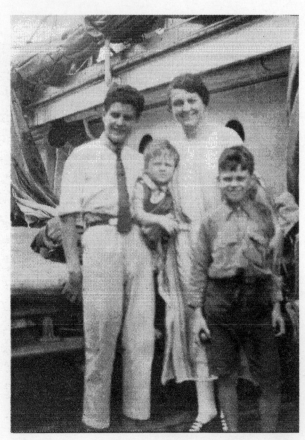

The Logue family on board the *Hobsons Bay*, 1924
Left to right: Laurie, Tony, Myrtle, Valentine

23rd November 1926

Dear Major Hodgson,

Following on a conversation with Her Royal Highness the Duchess of York at St.James Palace I would be very pleased if you would arrange an interview at 146 Harley Street,sometime during the coming week.

Yours very sincerely,

Major Patrick E.Hodgson
... Stanhope Gardens
S.W.7

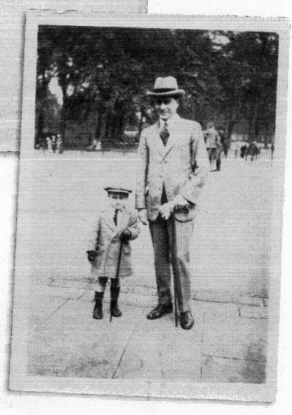

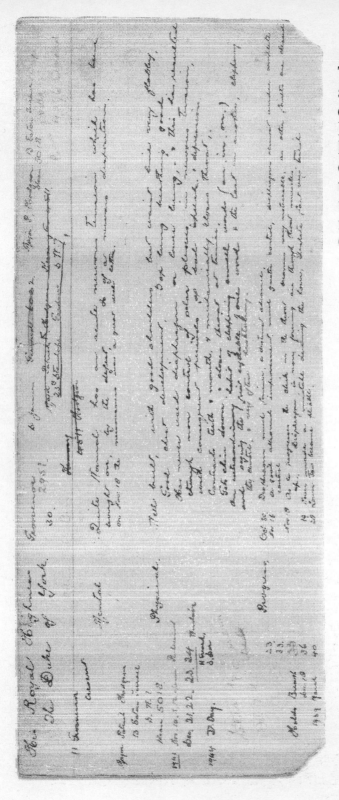

The appointment card on which Lionel noted his initial observations of the Duke after their first meeting in October 1926

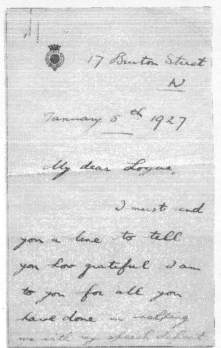

17 Buxton Street
W

January 5th 1927

My dear Logue,

I must send you a line to tell you how grateful I am to you for all you have done in helping me with my speech defect

I really do think you have given me a real good start in the way of getting over it & I am sure if I carry on with your exercises & instruction that I shall not go back. I am full of confidence for the trip anyhow. Again so very many thanks

I am
Yours very sincerely
Albert

Letter from the Duke expressing his gratitude at the progress he was already beginning to show at the start of his therapy. In the three months after his first interview, the Duke saw Lionel over fifty times

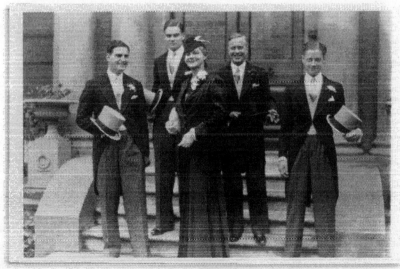

The Logue family dressed up in morning suits for Laurie's wedding day, in July 1936, on the steps of Beechgrove *Left to right: Laurie, Valentine, Myrtle, Lionel, Antony*

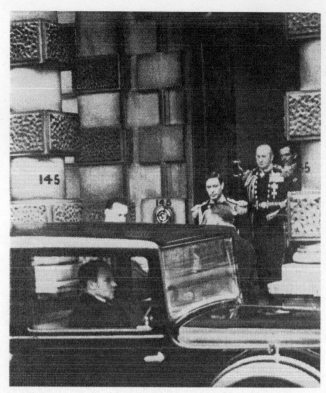

The Duke leaving 145 Piccadilly on his way to St James's Palace to take the Oath of Accession after the abdication of his brother, King Edward, 12 December 1936

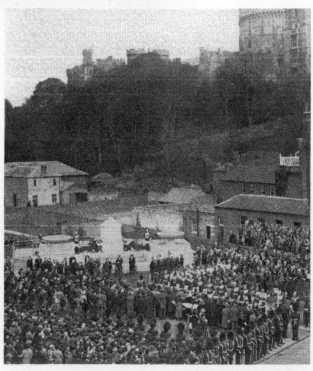

King George VI's first speech in public since his accession four months earlier, at the unveiling of the George V Memorial at Windsor on 23 April 1937

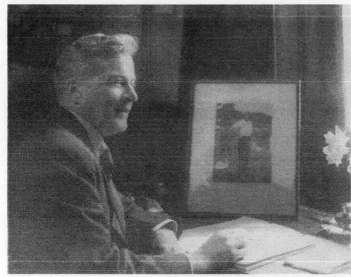

Lionel in his office at 146 Harley Street, with a portrait of Myrtle on his desk

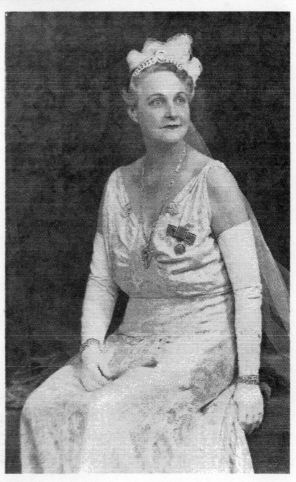

Myrtle in her Coronation gown

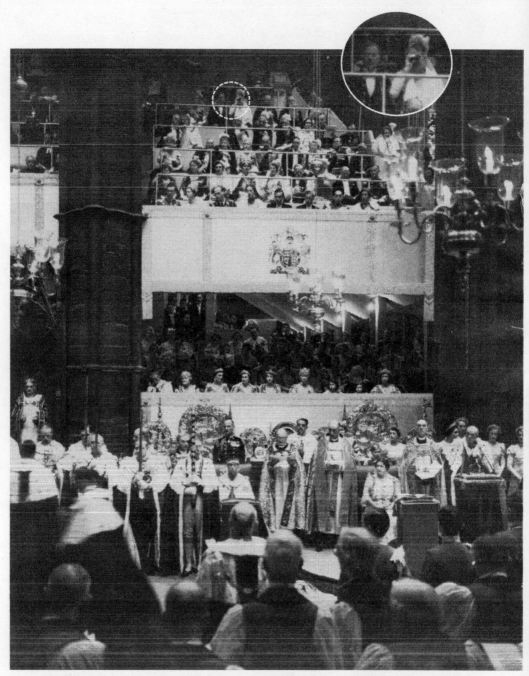

George VI's coronation on 12 May 1937. Logue and Myrtle are seated on the balcony above the Royal Box at Westminster Abbey

CHAPTER TEN

After the Coronation

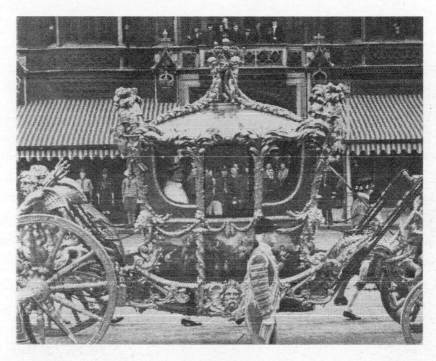

George VI and Queen Elizabeth on their way to
the state opening of Parliament, 12 October 1937

Both the coronation itself and the speech to the Empire that evening had been a triumph for the King—as next morning's newspapers noted. 'Slow, deliberate and clear, his voice betrayed no sign of fatigue,' commented the *Daily Telegraph*. A clergyman wrote to the *Daily Mail* from Manchester to express delight at 'the sound of the King's voice and the purity of his diction'. He continued: 'With all the depth of his father's voice, there is an additional softness which makes it even more impressive for the listener. I think it was the nearest approach to perfect "standard English" I have ever heard. There was no trace of anything which could be called accent.'

Those listening abroad were also pleasantly surprised by the fluency of the supposedly tongue-tied monarch. The compiler of the *Detroit Free Press*'s radio notes was baffled by what he had heard coming loud and clear over the ether from London. 'Now that the coronation is over, listeners are wondering what became of the speech impediment that King George VI was supposed to have,' he wrote. 'It wasn't apparent throughout the entire ceremony, and after hearing the new King deliver his address, many persons are classifying him with President Roosevelt as possessing a perfect radio voice.'

With the coronation behind him, the King was able to relax. He was still not completely cured of his speech impediment but, with Logue's assistance, he was gradually getting the better of it. Logue, meanwhile, suffering from what *Time* described as nervous exhaustion, was reported to have left London for a long rest. On his return, he helped the King prepare for the various speeches that were now becoming routine.

Although such speeches passed off fairly successfully, the King's staff were concerned about the effect his continuing speaking problems were having on him—and were forever on the lookout for ways of treating them. On 22 May Sir Alan 'Tommy' Lascelles, the King's assistant private secretary, wrote to Logue referring to a letter he had received from an A. J. Wilmott relating to correspondence in *The Times* about how forcing left-handed children to act as if they were right-handed could cause problems—among them speech impediments such as stammering.

In his reply, four days later, Logue notes how such practice can lead to a disorder—which may disappear if the patient is changed back to his natural hand. He stressed that it was too late for the King, however. 'After 10 years of age it becomes increasingly difficult to change the patient back again, and I have rarely heard of a case in which it has proved satisfactory in middle life.' Bizarrely, he suggested it might be possible to obtain 'temporary relief' from such a problem (often mistaken for a cure) by 'assuming an American or cockney accent', presumably since, as H. St John Rumsey, his fellow speech therapist, had argued, this would lead to a greater concentration on vowels rather than the dreaded consonants. It was clearly not an option for the King, though, even if some people had claimed to have heard something of a transatlantic twang in his elder brother's speech when he was monarch.

Logue's conclusion was that 'unfortunately in

the matter of Speech Defects, when so much depends on the temperament and individuality, a case can always be produced that can prove you are wrong. That is why I won't write a book.'

During a meeting on 20 July, Hardinge said the King was talking well but was overtired. Logue agreed, saying it was a shame he did not get more time to himself as he was overloaded. This impression was confirmed when he saw the King later that day: he seemed very drained and they had a long talk about his weak stomach and how it affected his speech.

'They certainly don't understand the King,' Logue wrote in his diary that same day. 'I, who know him so well, know just how much work he can stand up to and talk splendidly—give him too much work and make him too tired and it impacts on his weakest part—his speech. They are very foolish to overwork him. He will crash and they will only have themselves to blame.'[73]

The fear of such a crash was timely: the State Opening of Parliament was only a few months away and, although not nearly so much of an ordeal as the coronation, it would still pose a considerable challenge. There was also the question of Christmas and whether or not the King should follow the tradition established by his father of making a radio address to the people of the Empire.

The State Opening, at which the King would read out the programme of Neville Chamberlain's government (Chamberlain had become prime minister that May), was, of course, an unavoidable part of his duties as monarch. This did not prevent him worrying about it. He was preoccupied with how well George V had spoken to parliament in the past and was concerned he would fall short—as Logue noted after a meeting on 15 October when they had a run-through of the text. 'He is still worrying over the fact that his Father did this sort of thing so well,' Logue wrote in his diary. 'As I explained, it took his Father many years before he got in the excellent state he did.'

The King was actually making good progress with the text itself, which ran to 980 words and took him ten to twelve minutes to get through. But there was the further challenge of having to do so while wearing a heavy crown. When Logue arrived for a practice on the eve of the ceremony, he was surprised to see the King sitting on his chair running through the speech, with the crown perched on his head.

'He put it on so that he could find out how far he could bend to the left or right without it falling,' Logue wrote in his diary on 25 October. 'The crown fits so perfectly that there is no need to worry in the slightest.' After two successful run-throughs, the King put the crown away.

Both men were encouraged by his performance, even if the memory of his father continued to loom large. 'I have never heard him speak so well and have never known him so happy, or seen him look so well,' Logue wrote. 'If the King does well tomorrow, it will do him a tremendous amount of good. There is not the slightest need for him to do anything but well. It is only the inferiority complex about his Father, very nervous that is worrying him. His voice was beautiful tonight.'

The speech to parliament passed off

successfully, with that weekend's edition of the *Sunday Express* describing it as a triumph. 'He spoke slowly but there was no hesitation or stammer,' it said. 'Indeed, the words took on a dignity and actual beauty from the tempo that he had wisely imposed on himself.' The newspaper also noted how the King's confidence grew as the speech progressed, with him raising his eyes and glancing around the chamber. 'One does not need to be clairvoyant to understand what was passing through the Queen's mind,' it concluded. 'When the King had finished she could not keep from her eyes the pride of a woman in her husband.'

This still left the not inconsiderable matter of what to do about Christmas. On 25 December 1932 George V had begun what was to turn into a national tradition of the annual radio broadcast to the nation. Seated at a desk under the stairs in Sandringham, he had read out words written for him by Rudyard Kipling, the great imperial poet and author of *The Jungle Book*: 'I speak now from my home and from my heart to you all, to all my peoples throughout the Empire to men and women so cut off by the snows, the desert or the sea that only voices of the air can reach them, men and women of every race and colour who look to the Crown as the symbol of their union,' he declared.

George V made a further broadcast in 1935, in which he reflected not just on his Silver Jubilee but also on two other major royal events of the year: the marriage of his son Prince Henry, Duke of Gloucester, and the death of his sister Princess Victoria. The broadcasts, which were mildly, but not overly, religious in tone, were intended to cast

171

the monarch in the role of head of a great family spanning not just the United Kingdom but also the Empire—something his granddaughter, Queen Elizabeth II, was to strive to do during her more than half a century on the throne. Her Christmas messages, initially on radio and later on television, were to become an important part of the Christmas ritual for tens of millions of her subjects.

Neither George VI nor those around him saw it like that though. For him, the Christmas message was not a national tradition, merely something that his father had chosen to do, and the King had no desire to emulate him. The previous Christmas, with his elder brother's abdication only two weeks old, there had certainly been no expectation that he should speak. By December 1937, though, the situation was different and there was a clamour from the Empire in particular for the new King to make a broadcast. Thousands of letters began to arrive at Buckingham Palace urging him to speak.

The King was nevertheless still reluctant; part of this was the usual trepidation he continued to feel about any public speaking engagement, especially one that would require him to speak alone into a microphone to tens—maybe hundreds—of millions of people. He also seemed to feel that in making such a speech he would somehow be encroaching on his father's memory.

One solution, proposed by Hardinge at a meeting on 15 October, at which Logue was present, was that the King should instead read the lesson in church on Christmas morning. However, the idea was dropped because of concerns it might offend other denominations. The Palace was coming round to the idea that the King should read a short message to the Empire, and after a meeting on 4 November when Logue worked with the King on a couple more routine speeches, Hardinge showed him a rough draft which he proclaimed quite good.

Logue, meanwhile, had another concern. There were erroneous but persistent rumours that Princess Margaret, now aged seven, suffered from the same speech impediment as her father. Logue suggested to Hardinge that the next time she was in a news film, she should make a point of saying a few words—something like 'Come on, Mummy' or 'Where is Georgie?' or simply call the dog—'anything at all to prove that she can talk and lay for ever the rumour that she has a speech defect'.

November passed: a speech in honour of Léopold III, the King of the Belgians, went well. The King had also been apparently unfazed by an incident during the Remembrance Day ceremony at the Cenotaph when an ex-serviceman who had escaped from a mental asylum interrupted the two-minute silence with a shout of 'All this hypocrisy'.

When Logue met the King on 23 November, they had a long discussion about Christmas during which the King revealed he still hadn't quite made up his mind. One thing was clear, though: even if he did end up making a speech, it should not be seen as the reinstatement of an annual tradition. Logue didn't blame him and it was decided to make a final decision on the matter the following week. 'He is going down to Sandringham and then to the Duchy of Cornwall and will give it mature thought on the way,' Logue wrote. 'I should think

173

it would be a good thing to do a small broadcast this Xmas but certainly not every year.'

Despite the pressure of the decision weighing on him, the King was in a light-hearted mood, joking about official protocol at dinner as well as the problems of sitting ambassadors from hostile countries next to each other. He also laughed as he read Logue a rhyme about his brother and Wallis Simpson, chuckling when he got to the line, 'looked after State in day time and Mrs Wally at night'.

*　　*　　*

Christmas Day 1937 did not dawn very brightly, with an expectation of fog. Laurie Logue rose early and drove his father to Liverpool Street station, from where he was to take a train to Wolferton, the nearest station to Sandringham in north Norfolk, where the King and his family were spending Christmas.

Arrangements for Logue's journey had been left in the capable hands of C. J. Selway, the southern area passenger manager of the London & North Eastern Railway. Selway had sent Logue a third-class return rail ticket, together with a permit authorizing him to travel first class in both directions. A first-class smoking compartment had been reserved for him in the name of Mr George on the 9.40 train. The stationmaster came along to both wish him luck and make sure the right man had taken it. Logue was due to return to London on the 6.50p.m. train that evening.

The fog was patchy and they lost some time between Cambridge and Ely, but the train steamed

174

into King's Lynn only fifteen minutes late. Two stations down the line at Wolferton, a royal chauffeur was waiting on the platform for Logue. He picked up a large Royal Mail bag containing the mail for Sandringham, and they then set off for the estate.

'Nothing could have been more homely or sweeter than the hearty welcome they gave me,' recalled Logue. There were about twenty guests gathered in the reception room, gloriously carved in light oak with thirty-foot ceilings and a musician's gallery at one end. The King introduced him to everyone else before going in for lunch. Just as they were about to do so, a woman dressed in light blue moved up to his elbow, held out her hand and said, 'You are Mr Logue, I am very glad to meet you.' Logue bowed low over her outstretched hand. As he recorded in his diary, he had 'had the privilege of at last meeting one of the most wonderful women I have ever seen—Queen Mary'.

Before passing on to the dining room, guests stopped at the equerry's room where there was a flat leather model of the dining table, with white visiting cards showing the seating plan. Logue was pleased to see he was to sit between the Queen and the Duchess of Kent. The King was directly opposite.

The lunch, Logue recalled, 'was quite informal; jolly and lots of fun'. At 2.30 they went back to the beautiful reception room. But this was not just a social occasion: there was work to do. He joined the King in the study, the same room from which his late father had broadcast five years earlier, and they discussed the text and went through the

175

procedure to ensure everything was in place. They then went down the main hall, through the reception room and into the broadcasting room.

The oval table that George V had used to broadcast from had been pushed into a corner. In the centre of the room was a large desk with two microphones and the red light in the centre. The King, Logue found, was always much easier and less constrained in his speech when he could walk about—it made him laugh when he used to see posed photographs of him in the newspapers seated at a table.

Logue opened the window so there would be plenty of fresh air. They then joined R. H. Wood of the BBC who was in his own room. Quiet and fair haired, Wood probably knew more about the fledgling art of outside broadcasting than anyone else in Britain. It was Wood who had planned the installation of microphones for the coronation, and for that evening's speech. He had also been in charge of the technical side of George V's last broadcast, bringing along two microphones, cue lights and amplifiers as insurance against a breakdown. With him were six other men and all the paraphernalia of broadcasting: instruments, a telephone and a large loudspeaker through which they were to hear a record of the speech when it was relayed from Broadcasting House. The King was due to start talking at 3 p.m. precisely.

Despite the fog and gloom, everyone was in high spirits. Logue and the King went back to the microphone to try out the speech. As they did so, they could hear it booming back through the large radiogram in the room next door. So this was switched off and the rest of the royal family and their guests trooped up to the nursery to listen from there instead.

At five minutes to three, the King lit a cigarette and began to walk to and fro. Wood tried the red light to see it was working properly and they synchronized their watches. With one minute to go, the King threw his cigarette into the fireplace and stood with his hands behind his back, waiting. The red light flicked four times, and he stepped up to the microphone. The red light ceased for a moment and then came back on full, and he began to speak in a beautifully modulated voice.

'Many of you will remember the Christmas broadcasts of former years, when my father spoke to his peoples, at home and overseas, as the revered head of a great family . . .'

He was speaking too quickly: close to a hundred words a minute, rather than the eighty-five that Wood had wanted. He also had trouble with one of the words, running on to it too quickly.

'His words brought happiness into the homes and into the hearts of listeners all over the world,' the King continued. Logue was pleased to note that he was pulling himself up.

Then, high up in the speech—an inclusion that was to be noted by the newspapers—came the insistence that this was to be a one-off rather than a tradition: 'I cannot aspire to take his place—nor do I think that you would wish me to carry on, unvaried, a tradition so personal to him.'

The King continued at the same pace, sweetly towards the end, when he paused. After precisely three minutes and twenty seconds, it was all over. 'Just a shade too long on two words through trying to get too much of an emphasis,' Logue recorded.

But to the King, he said: 'May I be the first to congratulate you, Sire, on your first Christmas Broadcast.' The King shook his hand, gave what Logue described as 'that lovely schoolboy grin of his', and said, 'Let's go inside.'

They went back into the reception room where the royal family and guests were thronging down from the nursery. They crowded round the King and they, too, congratulated him. It was now 3.20 and the royal family and visitors began to disperse: some went to their rooms; others went out for a short walk. The King, his wife and mother went back into Wood's room to wait and hear the broadcast played back.

Queen Mary, aged seventy, was as interested as a schoolgirl in all the paraphernalia and, after shaking hands with all the men, had the instruments explained to her. Then the telephone rang. Wood took the call and said, 'London is now ready to play it back to us, your Majesty.' Queen Mary sat in front of the microphone and Logue stood with his hand on the chair. The King was leaning against the wall, and the Queen, her face animated and flushed, was standing in the doorway.

Then the opening bars of 'God save the King' came through and they heard the speech back again. When it was over, Queen Mary thanked them all and asked Wood: 'Was all this done when my late husband broadcasted and were all you gentlemen here?'

'Yes, your Majesty,' replied Wood.

'And I knew nothing about it,' replied Mary, rather sadly as it seemed to Logue.

As they passed through the microphone room,

178

her daughter-in-law, Queen Elizabeth, stopped Logue and, putting her hand on his shoulder, said: 'Mr Logue, I do not know that Bertie and myself can ever thank you enough for what you have done for him. Just look at him now. I do not think I have ever known him so light-hearted and happy.'

Logue was overcome with emotion, and it was as much as he could do to stop tears trickling down his cheeks. They then walked through into the reception room and he, the King and the Queen sat in front of the fire for nearly an hour, talking through the many things that had happened in the seven months since the coronation.

Just before it was time for tea, the King stood up. 'Oh, Logue, I want to speak to you,' he said. Logue followed him to the library. He took from his desk a picture of himself, the Queen and the little princesses in their coronation robes, which they both had autographed, as well as a box. Inside was a beautiful replica of a silver tobacco box, and a pair of gold sleeve links in black enamel with the royal arms and Crown.

Logue was too overcome to say much, but the King patted him on the back. 'I do not know that I can ever thank you enough for all that you have done for me,' he said.

Tea was another informal meal: the Queen was at one end of the table and Lady May Cambridge at the other. Afterwards, they all went down to the big decorated ballroom, where Logue was to receive an insight into the highly organized ritual of royal present-giving. In the centre of the room was a large Christmas tree stretching up to the roof, beautifully decorated. All around the room huge trestle tables had been put up, covered in white paper. They were about three feet wide and divided every three feet by a blue ribbon, giving everyone a space three feet square. Each space was marked with a name tag, starting with the King and Queen, and inside was that person's presents.

The King had given the Queen a lovely sapphire coronet, but Logue was struck by the simplicity of both the whole procedure and the other presents, especially those given to the children. Then they all played 'Ring a Ring o' Roses' with the two princesses and the other royal children.

For Logue, the time went by almost in a dream until at 6.30 Commander Lang, the equerry, pointed out that if he was going to make his train back to London he would have to set off presently, especially because of the fog. Earlier that afternoon, the Queen had offered to Logue to stay the night if he wanted, but he was reluctant to outstay his welcome. There was also the matter of his own guests waiting for him back at his home in Sydenham.

In the meantime the King, his wife and mother had gone into the nearby long room to hand out presents to staff and people on the estate, but when the equerry whispered to them that Logue was leaving, they broke off to bid him farewell.

So Logue bowed over the two queens' hands and they both thanked him sweetly for what he had done, and then the King shook his hand and said how much he appreciated his having sacrificed Christmas dinner on his behalf. 'Anyhow,' he said, 'as there is no dining car on the train I have arranged for a hamper to be left for you.'

Outside it was now terribly foggy, but the driver

somehow made it to Wolferton in good time and Logue was soon on the train back to London, accompanied by a hamper containing a beautiful Christmas dinner with the King's compliments. Despite the fog, the train pulled into Liverpool Street three minutes ahead of schedule. Laurie, who had left his own Christmas dinner, was waiting to bring his father home. By 10.45 Logue was receiving another welcome in his own home where all the guests seemed well and happy. And so ended what he described as 'one of the most wonderful days I have ever had in my life'.

*   *   *

Myrtle did not join her husband at Sandringham. That spring, she had begun to suffer from an inflamed gall bladder, and on 5 July was operated on. The surgeon removed fourteen stones, 'enough to make a rockery', as she put it in a letter to her brother Rupert. She spent more than three weeks in hospital before she was discharged, but suffered a relapse ten days later, when a splinter of stone left behind began to move. As she lurched from crisis to crisis, Lionel was distraught at the possibility of losing the woman who had been by his side for most of his adult life. That March, they had celebrated their thirtieth wedding anniversary —'a terrible time to spend with one woman and yet looking back there are few things that I would like altered,' he wrote. 'It has been a very wonderful time, and she has always been behind me to give me the extra little shove I want.'

Myrtle's doctors wanted to spare her the British winter and prescribed a few months in Australia to

181

recuperate. She set off on 4 November 1937 from Southampton as one of the 499 passengers aboard the 8,640-ton *Jervis Bay* of the Aberdeen and Commonwealth Line. She arrived at Fremantle, in Western Australia, on 5 December, spent four weeks in Perth and then continued eastwards across the country. She wasn't due to return to Britain until the following April.

It was the first time Myrtle had been home since she and Lionel had left more than a decade earlier. Thanks to her husband's success and proximity to the monarch, she was treated as a celebrity: parties, concerts and recitals were thrown in her honour, and she was a guest of the Governor of Victoria, Lord Huntingfield, and his wife at Government House. Journalists flocked to interview the woman described as the 'wife of King George's voice specialist', and the society columns of the newspapers recorded where she went, whom she met and what she was wearing. Myrtle seemed only too happy to bask in the reflected glory, even though she suffered a few health scares along the way—at one stage she was so bad they thought they would have to take her to Adelaide in an ambulance, but she rallied until she was 'a bit yellow but able to carry on'.

In one newspaper interview, published under the headline 'Australians Thrive in London', Myrtle painted a rosy picture of the life that she and her compatriots enjoyed in the mother country, noting how many of them had achieved prominence in London. 'I put it down to their self-confidence and freedom from fear,' she declared. 'They are most capable and adaptable, and seem to fall on their feet in every walk of life.' She also described how her own 'lovely home' on Sydenham Hill had become a 'calling-point' for Australians visiting Britain.

While Lionel was always discreet when it came to talking about his work, his wife couldn't stop herself from discussing the King, boasting how he had personally invited her and her husband to his coronation. The monarch, she told one interviewer, is 'the hardest worker in the world', a man with 'enormous vitality and strength' that enables him to cope with his workload. She spoke warmly of his 'particularly happy smile—a grin you could call it' and his 'wonderful sense of humour'.

'If all my husband's patients showed the grit and determination of the King all his cures would be 100 per cent,' she told another interviewer. 'His Majesty frequently comes to our house—he is most charming. So are the Princesses, who are completely unspoilt, although Margaret Rose is the more joyous—Elizabeth has rather more sense of responsibility.

'They both speak beautifully and are simple and unassuming,' she added. 'My husband goes to the Palace every night now, and always the little Princesses come in to say "Goodnight, Daddy".'[74]

Quite what Myrtle's husband thought about such indiscretions is not clear. His disapproval cannot have been that strong, however, since the newspaper cuttings in which his wife was quoted were all diligently glued in his scrapbook.

CHAPTER ELEVEN

The Path to War

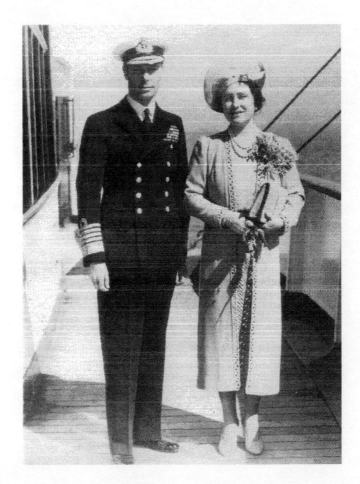

George VI and Queen Elizabeth en route to
Canada, 1939

While Myrtle was making her triumphal progress through Australia, Europe was moving inexorably towards war. For several years, as part of his pursuit of *Lebensraum*, Hitler had been turning his attention to the area along the German border occupied largely by German-speaking people. In 1935, following a plebiscite, the Saar region was united with Germany. Then in early 1938 came *Anschluss* with Austria. This left Czechoslovakia, a tempting target with its substantial ethnic German population, who formed a majority in some districts in the Sudetenland. The landlocked country was also hemmed in on three sides. When, in the spring and summer of 1938, some Sudeten Germans began to agitate for autonomy or even union with Germany, Hitler took it as the excuse he needed to act.

Czechoslovakia had a well-trained army, but its government knew that it would prove no match for the might of the Nazi war machine. The Czechs needed the support of Britain and France, but London and Paris were about to hang them out to dry. That September, Chamberlain met Hitler at his lair at Berchtesgaden, where it was agreed that Germany could annexe the Sudetenland, provided a majority of its inhabitants voted in favour in a plebiscite. Czechoslovakia's remaining rump would then receive international guarantees of its independence. But when Chamberlain flew back to see the Nazi leader in Bad Godesberg, near Bonn, on 22 September, Hitler brushed aside the previous agreement.

Chamberlain was still in Germany when Logue

met the King the next day. The reason for their meeting was a speech the King had to make for the launch of the *Queen Elizabeth*, on 27 September. He was understandably preoccupied by the worsening international situation and wanted to know from Logue what ordinary people thought about the prospect of war. The King, like so many of his generation, had been so appalled by the slaughter of the First World War that he seemed to consider anything—even appeasement of the Nazi leader—preferable to another all-out conflict. 'You would be astonished, Logue, at the number of people who wish to plunge this country into war, without counting the cost,' he told him.

Even if the King had thought otherwise, there was little he could have done about it: the influence of the monarch had declined considerably over the previous thirty years. In the first decade of the century, his grandfather Edward VII had been actively involved in foreign policy, helping pave the way for the Entente Cordiale with France in 1904. George VI, by contrast, would have little scope for changing the policies being pursued by Chamberlain and his ministers.

And so, in the early hours of 30 September, Chamberlain and his French counterpart Edouard Daladier, together with Hitler and Mussolini, signed what became known as the Munich Agreement allowing Germany to annexe the Sudetenland. On his return to London, Chamberlain waved a copy of the agreement to jubilant crowds at Heston airport in west London, stating his conviction that it meant 'peace for our time'. Many believed him.

Munich did not prevent war, however; it merely

188

postponed it. In the months that followed Logue continued to meet the King, becoming a frequent visitor to Buckingham Palace; there could be no more question of him visiting Logue in Harley Street as he had done when he was Duke of York.

The first immediate challenge for the King was the speech he was due to make for the State Opening of Parliament, set for 8 November 1938. He was also preparing for an important journey— a trip of more than a month to Canada, starting in early May 1939. This was the first by a reigning British monarch and was, if anything, even more important than his voyage to Australia and New Zealand more than a decade earlier that had prompted the beginning of his association with Logue. In the speech he was to confirm that while in Canada he would be accepting an invitation from President Franklin D. Roosevelt to make a short private visit across the border to the United States. The visits were not just about strengthening Britain's bonds with the two North American powers. It was also a deliberate attempt to shore up sympathy there ahead of the conflict with Nazi Germany that now seemed inevitable.

Logue had been asked to go to the Palace at 6 p.m. on 3 November to run through the speech with the King. He arrived fifteen minutes early and dropped in on Alexander Hardinge, who showed him the text. As he read it, Logue was pleased to see the King would be accepting Roosevelt's invitation. 'I consider it the greatest gesture for world peace that has ever been made,' he wrote in his diary. 'Of course a lot of US citizens will argue and say it is a political dodge but they read either politics or money into everything.'

189

While he was there reading, the King's assistant private secretary Eric Mieville came in, and he and Hardinge started to discuss at length the wisdom or otherwise of the King taking representatives of the Court with him to Canada. Unable to decide, they turned to Logue for his opinion 'as a colonial'. Logue had fond memories from his childhood of the visit to Adelaide paid by King George V, when he was still Duke of York. 'The more pageantry the better,' he told them. 'This they accepted and the Lord Chamberlain will probably never know that it was the opinion of colonial Lionel Logue that got him included in the Canadian Tour.'

The King looked tired, understandably perhaps, since he had got up at four o'clock that morning to go duck shooting at Sandringham. To Logue's eyes, he seemed in fairly good form, though. They went through the speech twice: the first time it took them thirteen minutes; by the second, they had got it down to eleven. It was written in the usual difficult language, though, and they fixed two other appointments for further preparation. Before he left, a few minutes before seven o'clock, Princess Margaret, who was then almost eight, came in to say goodnight to her father. 'It is very beautiful to see these two playing together,' thought Logue. 'He never takes his eyes off her when she is in the room.'

Logue met the King again on the morning of the State Opening for a final run-through: 'A good effort, despite the fact that the redundancy of words is dreadful,' he wrote in his diary. 'It took 11 minutes exactly and it will be interesting to know how long he takes to deliver it.' Logue couldn't go to parliament himself, but Captain Charles Lambe, one of the King's officials who was going to be present in the chamber, promised to time the speech and call him immediately afterwards. Lambe reported later that it had taken thirteen minutes and there had been four hesitations.

*   *   *

To the relief of Logue—and even more so of the King himself—it was decided that there would be no Christmas message that year; the previous one had been a one-off, delivered only because it had been coronation year. Any such relief was short lived, however: during his visit to North America, the King would have to make a number of speeches, the most important of which was in Winnipeg on 24 May, Empire Day. First marked in 1902 on the birthday of Queen Victoria, who had died the previous year, the day was intended to remind children what it meant to be 'sons and daughters of a glorious Empire'. At a time of great international tension such as this, it provided an opportunity for a display of solidarity on the part of the members of the Empire towards the mother country.

All these speeches necessarily meant a number of sessions for the King with Logue. A letter sent from the Palace on 10 March, for example, confirmed appointments at the Palace for the 16th, 17th and 20th. Such frequent visits meant Logue was also beginning to see more of the King's family. During the first of those three appointments, Princess Margaret Rose again interrupted them—captivating Logue with her charm, just as her mother always did. 'What a dear mature little woman she is with her bright eyes that do not miss a thing,' he noted in his diary. 'She had just come from a dancing lesson and showed us how in doing the last steps of the Highland fling her little shoes scraped her legs and after demonstrating it she [asked that] "something be done about it".'

The following month, Logue encountered the formidable figure of Queen Mary, the Queen Mother, who was by then in her early seventies. As he was walking down the curved corridor on his way to the King, he saw around the corner that one of the footmen was standing stiffly to attention. A few steps later, he noticed two women coming towards him, one of whom was walking with the aid of a stick. Logue's heart leapt into his mouth as he suddenly realized who she was.

'I backed into the wall, and bowed, they got opposite me, and then stopped—and I was afraid my heart was going to do the same,' Logue recorded in his diary, in the rather breathless tone he reserved for his encounters with royal women. 'The Queen approached me slowly—and as she put her hand out said, "I know you—you came to Sandringham. Of course, you are Logue, I am very glad to see you again."'

Later, when he told the King how impressed he had been that his mother had recognized him, the King replied, 'Yes she is very wonderful.'

The King and Queen were due to leave on 5 May 1939, taking the Canadian Pacific liner RMS *Empress of Australia* on what would be a twelve-day voyage across the north Atlantic. The afternoon before, Logue was summoned to the

192

Palace. He gave Tommy Lascelles, who was to accompany them, advice on how to help the King get ready to broadcast. One of the important tips was that, contrary to the impression given by all the photographs of him sitting in front of the microphone, he actually preferred to stand. On this occasion (just as had been the case with the Australian trip) there was no question of Logue being included in the Royal party—nor did he want to be. 'My wonderful patient goes on wonderfully well, and should have a marvellous time in Canada,' he wrote to his brother-in-law Rupert. 'Don't think there is any need for me to go.'

Then, a few minutes later, the message came down: 'Mr Logue wanted', and he was shown into the King's presence. As Logue recalled, he was too tired to stand up and go through his speeches, but he was smiling and seemed quite happy. They were working together on the text of a Quebec speech when a hidden door in the wall opened and in came the Queen, looking striking in brown, accompanied by the two princesses.

Elizabeth and Margaret begged that, as it was their last night with their parents, they should be allowed to stay up and go to the swimming pool. The Queen added her voice and, after many pleas of 'do, Daddy it's our last night', the King gave in, provided they were finished by 6.30.

He then turned to Logue and said, 'Tell them the time you dived on the shark.' So Logue told the story of how when he was a boy of five or so living in Brighton, on the coast of South Australia, he and the other children used to jump out of bed first thing in the morning and run to the jetty, shedding their pyjamas as they went, in the race to be first into the water.

On this particular morning, the young Logue was first and he dived off the end of the little jetty with a joyous shout—into the sparkling, crystal clear water. 'As I turned over in the air, there below me in about ten feet of water, fast asleep, was a small shark,' he went on. 'I couldn't go back, and I struck the water with a frightful slap and then struck out for the landing stage, expecting every instant to lose a leg. The unfortunate shark, probably more scared than I was, I have no doubt was by this time, five miles down the Gulf.' As Logue told the story, the princesses, their eyes open wide and their hands clasped, gazed at him enthralled.

Once the two girls had gone off to the pool, Logue shook hands with the Queen and wished her a good trip and safe return. 'Well, I hope we don't work too hard anyhow,' she replied. 'We are looking forward to coming home already.'

Alone with the King again, Logue had him go through the speeches one more time. 'The King did them splendidly,' he noted in his diary. 'If he does not get too tired I am certain he will do wonderfully well. As I was going, I wished him all sorts of good luck and he thanked me and said, many thanks Logue, for all your trouble, I am *very* lucky to have a man who understands voices and speeches so well.'

The journey to Canada was not without its dramas: the ice field had come much further south than usual during the winter and there was thick fog, and the ship only narrowly avoided an iceberg. As someone on board pointed out to the

194

unfortunate captain, it had been near this point during a similar season in 1912 that the *Titanic* had come to grief.

The King and Queen landed in Quebec on 17 May, a few days later than planned, and embarked on a packed schedule that took them across the country. At almost every point they received an enthusiastic welcome. As one Provincial premier told Lascelles: 'You can go home and tell the Old Country that any talk they may hear about Canada being isolationist after to-day is just nonsense.'[75] A week later came the Empire Day speech, which was broadcast back in Britain at 8 p.m. Logue listened to it and afterwards sent a telegram to Lascelles, who was by then aboard the royal train in Winnipeg.

'Empire Broadcast tremendous success, voice beautiful, resonant speed, eighty minimum atmospheres. Please convey congratulations loyal wishes to His Majesty. Regards Logue'.

The American leg of their journey, which began on the evening of 9 June, was if anything of even greater importance for the King: members of the royal family had visited the United States before, but this was the first time a reigning British sovereign had set foot on the country's soil. A royal red carpet was spread on the station platform at Niagara Falls, in New York State, as the blue and silver royal train crossed the border and the King and Queen were met by Cordell Hull, the secretary of state, and his wife.

President Roosevelt was keenly aware of symbolism when he issued the invitation. If the Canadian leg of the King and Queen's trip had been intended to underline Commonwealth

195

solidarity, the King's presence south of the 49th parallel would offer powerful proof of the strength of Britain's friendship with the United States.

The reaction to the royal couple on the streets of Washington was extraordinary. An estimated 600,000 people walked the royal route from Union Station, past the Capitol, down Pennsylvania Avenue to the White House, despite temperatures that hit 94°F. 'In the course of a long life I have seen many important events in Washington, but never have I seen a crowd such as lined the whole route between the Union Station and the White House,' Eleanor Roosevelt, the President's wife, wrote in her diary, adding, of the royal couple, 'They have a way of making friends, these young people'.[76]

For the King, the highpoint of the visit was the twenty-four hours that he and the Queen spent at Hyde Park, Roosevelt's country house on the bank of the Hudson River in Dutchess County, New York. Although the Royal Standard flew from the portico, the men put all formality aside and spoke frankly about the worsening international situation and its impact on their respective countries.

Both couples also hit it off on a personal level, drinking cocktails and enjoying a picnic lunch at which the King took off his tie, drank beer and sampled that great American delicacy, the hot dog. The Roosevelts, noted *Time* magazine, had 'developed a father-&-motherly feeling towards this nice young couple'. The King and Queen seemed rather to enjoy it. 'They are such a charming & united family, and living so like English people when they come to their country house,' the Queen wrote to her mother-in-law.[77]

Wheeler-Bennett, the King's official biographer, speculated that Roosevelt, who was confined to a wheelchair by polio, and the King, with his difficulties in speaking, had been brought closer to one another by 'that unspoken bond which unites those who have triumphed over physical disability'.

*   *   *

The King and Queen set off for home on 15 June from Halifax, aboard the liner *Empress of Britain*. There was no doubting the importance of the contribution the visit had made not just to Britain's relationship with the New World, but also to the King's own self-esteem—a point noted by the press on both sides of the Atlantic. 'The trip nowhere had more influence than on George VI himself,' noted *Time* four days later. 'Two years ago he took on his job at a few hours' notice, having expected to play a quiet younger brother role to brother Edward all his life. Pressmen who followed him around the long loop from Quebec to Halifax were struck by the added poise and self-confidence that George drew from the ordeal.'

The theme was picked up later by the King's official biographer. The trip 'had taken him out of himself, had opened up for him wider horizons and introduced him to new ideas', he noted. 'It marked the end of his apprenticeship as a monarch, and gave him self-confidence and assurance.'[78]

This self-confidence had been reflected in the speeches that the King had made during the visit. 'I have never heard the King—or indeed few other people—speak so effectively, or so movingly,'

Lascelles wrote to Mackenzie King, the Canadian prime minister. 'One or two passages obviously stirred him so deeply that I feared he might break down. This spontaneous feeling heightened the force of the speech considerably . . . The last few weeks, culminating in his final effort today, have definitely established him as a first-class public speaker.'[79]

The King's British subjects had a chance to appreciate his newfound confidence at a lunch at the Guildhall on Friday 23 June, the day after he and the Queen returned to London to a tumultuous welcome. The King had cabled Logue from the ship to be at the Palace at 11.15. He arrived early enough to have a brief word with Hardinge, who told him the King was tired but in great form.

As always, the King seemed a little nervous to Logue, but he soon relaxed and broke into his characteristic grin as they spent a couple of minutes talking about the trip. 'He was most interested in Roosevelt—a most delightful man he called him,' Logue wrote. They ran through the speech, which Logue thought too long; as ever straying beyond the mere words to the content itself, he also made clear his belief that it should contain more references to the American part of the trip. The King noted his advice, but with the speech due to be delivered only a few hours later, it was a bit late for either of them to do anything about it.

Some seven hundred of the great and good were invited to the Guildhall, where they were treated to an eight-course lunch, washed down with two brands of 1928 champagne and vintage port. 'It is a great pity that a colour film was not made of the scene,' commented the *Daily Express*. 'It would have preserved for posterity a close-up of the entire executive power of Britain, tightly packed on a few square yards of blue carpet.'

Speaking with great emotion, the King described how the visit had underlined the strength of links between Britain and Canada. 'I saw everywhere not only the mere symbol of the British Crown; I saw also, flourishing strongly as they do here, the institutions which have developed, century after century, beneath the aegis of that Crown,' he told his audience, who interrupted him several times with loud cheers.

Logue, who listened to the speech on the radio, was impressed. Lascelles called him at 4.15 'to say how pleased everyone was with the speech, *particularly the King*'.

The verdict of the press was also positive. The *Daily Express*'s William Hickey column described it as 'an admirable, shapely speech' with personal touches that gave the impression the King had composed it himself. It was well delivered, too. 'The King has improved so enormously in this respect since the early days of his reign that one is not now conscious of any impediment,' the newspaper noted, adding that he had developed the orator's art of leaving just enough time for the loud cheers that punctuated his speech.

The following month the King expressed his own reaction to the growing praise for his skills as an orator in his reply to a letter of congratulation from his old friend Sir Louis Greig. 'It was a change from the old days when speaking, I felt, was "hell",' he wrote.[80]

CHAPTER TWELVE

'Kill the Austrian House Painter'

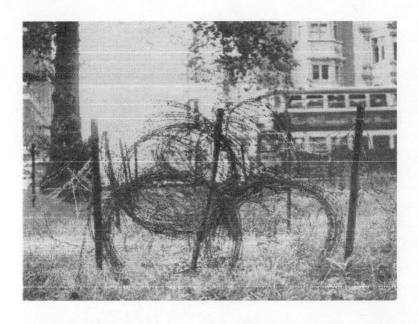

Green Park took on a very different aspect during
World War Two

On the morning of Sunday 3 September 1939 the inevitable finally happened: Sir Nevile Henderson, the British ambassador to Berlin, delivered a final note to the German government stating that unless the country withdrew the troops it had sent into Poland two days earlier by eleven o'clock that day, Britain would declare war. No such undertaking was given, and at 11.15 Neville Chamberlain went on the radio to announce, in sorrowful and heartfelt tones, that Britain was now at war with Germany. France followed suit a few hours later.

The House of Commons met on a Sunday for the first time in its history to hear Chamberlain's report. One of the prime minister's first acts was a reshuffle that brought Winston Churchill back into government as First Lord of the Admiralty, the post he had held during the First World War. Anthony Eden, who had resigned in protest over the prime minister's policy of appeasement in February 1938, returned as secretary for the dominions. Chamberlain was now seventy years of age and already suffering from the cancer that would kill him little more than a year later—but not before he had been forced to resign, ceding the premiership to Churchill who was five years his junior.

There had been a feeling throughout that sweltering summer that war was imminent. The announcement on 22 August of a non-aggression pact between Germany and the Soviet Union brought the conflict one step closer, by giving Hitler a free hand to invade Poland and then turn his forces on the West. Three days later, Britain signed a treaty with the government in Warsaw pledging to come to its assistance if it were attacked. Chamberlain nevertheless continued to negotiate with Hitler, even though he turned down the King's offer to write a personal letter to the Nazi leader. For many people, the worst thing was the uncertainty.

On 28 August Logue was summoned to the Palace. Alexander Hardinge, exceptionally, was there in his shirtsleeves. It was uncomfortably hot—the kind of weather Logue would have expected back home in Australia rather than in his adoptive nation. 'One of the most stifling and unpleasant days that I can ever remember, reminded me more of Sydney or Ceylon than any day in England,' he wrote in his diary.

The King and his aides seemed as frustrated as everyone else in the country about the lack of resolution of the crisis—as Logue noted. 'I went into the King and his first words were "Hello Logue, can you tell me, are we at war?"' he wrote. 'I said I didn't know and he said, "You don't know, the Prime Minister doesn't know, and I don't know." He is greatly worried, and said the whole thing is so damned unreal. If we only knew which way it was going to be.' By the time Logue went home, however, he was convinced that 'war is just around the corner'.

Then, on 1 September, German troops moved into Poland. 'Britain Gives Last Warning,' screamed the front page headline of the *Daily Express* the following morning. 'Either stop hostilities and withdraw German troops from Poland or we will go to war.' The smaller sub-headline immediately below provided the answer:

204

'An ultimatum we will reject, says Berlin.'

Over the last few months the government had been preparing Britain and its civilian population for war—and what was expected to be heavy bombing of its major cities. Some 827,000 schoolchildren were evacuated to the country, alongside just over 100,000 teachers and their helpers, from London and other urban areas. A further 524,000 children below school age left with their mothers. The cities themselves were protected with air-raid sirens and barrage balloons; windows were to be covered with black-out paper. Trenches were dug in parks and air-raid shelters. Those with gardens of their own dug holes in which they erected corrugated-iron Anderson shelters, covering the structure over with the earth they had removed. It was recommended they dig down at least three feet.

One of the greatest fears was of chemical warfare. Poison gas had been used to horrific effect in the trenches during the First World War and there was concern that the Germans might use it against civilians in this conflict. By the outbreak of war, some 38 million black rubber gas masks had been handed out, accompanied by a propaganda campaign. 'Hitler will send no warning—so always carry your gas mask,' read one advertisement. Those caught without one risked a fine.

The Logues, like everyone else, were preparing for the worst. Starting on the night of 1 September, street lights were turned off and everyone had to cover up their windows at night to make it more difficult for German bombers to find their targets. Tony, their youngest, an athletic young man with

205

wavy brown hair who was soon to celebrate his nineteenth birthday, came back from the local library bearing a sheet of black-out paper and embarked on making all the windows lightproof. Fortunately all the main rooms had shutters—Myrtle hated them and had long contemplated ripping them out but was now rather glad she hadn't.

There wasn't enough black-out paper to do all the windows so Tony had left one uncovered in the bathroom. It didn't seem much of a concern but that evening, a few minutes after Myrtle went in to clean her teeth before going to bed, there was a knock on the front door. She opened it to two air-raid precaution wardens who told her in courteous tones that she should turn out the light. Sleeping in a blacked-out room was also an unfamiliar experience: Myrtle felt like a 'chrysalis in a cocoon of semi-gloom'.

The family had a more immediate problem: Therese, their devoted cook, who had lived in London for the previous ten years, was originally from Bavaria. 'Oh Madam, I am caught—it is too late to get away,' she told Myrtle, tears streaming down her cheeks. That afternoon they had turned on the radio, only to hear an alarming notice of general mobilization. Therese rang the German embassy and was told there was a last train leaving at ten o'clock the next morning, and she rushed away to pack.

In the Logue household, as elsewhere in the country, the sense of apprehension was leavened by some lighter moments. 'The charwoman turned a tense situation into one of great comedy,' Logue recalled. 'Her boy Ernie was taken to the country yesterday, and as she went downstairs she said "Thank God my Ernie has been excavated."'

However unwelcome the prospect of fighting another war, only just over two decades after the end of the last one, Chamberlain's declaration of 3 September meant the people of Britain at least now knew where they stood. 'A marvellous relief after all our tension,' wrote Logue. 'The universal desire is to kill the Austrian house painter.' The King expressed similar sentiments in his own diary, which he was to keep dutifully for the next seven and a half years. 'As eleven o'clock struck that fateful morning I had a certain feeling of relief that those 10 anxious days of intensive negotiations with Germany over Poland, which at moments looked favourable, with Mussolini working for peace as well, were over,' he wrote.[81]

Myrtle, meanwhile, was preoccupied with more practical matters: she made 10lb of damson jam and 8lb of beans to salt down. War or no war, they had to eat. Laurie and his wife Josephine—or Jo, as she was known in the family—were also there. Myrtle was worried about them: Jo was expecting their first child (Lionel and Myrtle's first grandchild) at the end of that month. As Myrtle wrote in the diary that she was now keeping, she hoped that Jo would be 'excavated' too.

A few minutes after Chamberlain had finished speaking, the unfamiliar wail of air-raid sirens could be heard across London. Logue called Tony, who was in the garage mending his bicycle, and they began to close all the shutters. From their window they could see the barrage balloon going up—it was, Logue noted, a 'wonderful sight'. A few miles away in Buckingham Palace, the King

207

and Queen were also surprised to hear the ghastly wailing of the sirens. The two of them looked at each other and said, 'it can't be'. But it was, and with their hearts beating hard they went down to the shelter in the basement. There, in the Queen's words, they 'felt stunned & horrified, and sat waiting for bombs to fall'.[82]

There were no bombs that particular night, and about half an hour later the all-clear went up. The royal couple, like others fortunate enough to have access to a shelter, returned to their homes. It was to be the first of many such false alarms as the much feared air raids on London were not to start in earnest until the Blitz almost exactly a year later.

The first night of the war started like any other. The only difference Myrtle noticed was there were no programmes on the radio; they just played records. Then at 3 a.m. came another air-raid warning and they hurried down to the stuffy basement. 'The only feeling is one of irritation,' she wrote in her diary. 'It is strange how things work out—no panic, no fear only plain mad at being disturbed.'

The blackout was into its third night and continuing to cause chaos in a city unused to total darkness. The casualty departments of the hospitals were full—not with those hit by enemy fire, but instead with people who had been run over by cars whose headlights had been partially dimmed, broken their legs while stepping off trains onto nonexistent platforms or sprained their ankles stumbling over unseen kerbs. St George's, where Valentine was a resident surgical officer after qualifying three years earlier, was no

208

exception: that first day of the war he was up all night operating on people who had come to grief on the streets of London.

*   *   *

Now war had been declared, Logue knew he would have an important role to play at the King's side. On the previous Monday, 25 August, he had been called by Hardinge. 'Hold yourself in readiness to come to the Palace,' he had told him. Logue did not need to ask why. He was ready day and night although, as he told Hardinge, much as he wanted to see and speak to the King again, he sincerely hoped that he wouldn't be sent for—since he knew only too well what it would mean.

At midday on 3 September came the call he had been dreading. Eric Mieville, who had been assistant private secretary to the King since 1937, rang to say that the King would broadcast to the nation at 6 p.m. and asked Logue to come and see him. Laurie drove him into the city and he was at the Palace by 5.20 p.m.

As they made their way towards London, everything looked normal except for the sun shining on the blimps turning them a 'lovely silvery blue'. After dropping off his father at the Palace, Laurie turned back home at once so he could be there in time to listen to the broadcast. Logue left his hat, umbrella and gas mask in the Privy Purse Hall and mounted the stairs.

The King received Logue in his private study, rather than the room they normally used, which was being prepared for the post-broadcast photograph. He was dressed in an admiral's

209

uniform, with all his ribbons, and they ran through the speech. Its message, according to his official biographer, was 'a declaration of simple faith in simple beliefs . . . which gave encouragement, as perhaps nothing else could, to the British peoples in the face of the struggle which lay ahead, and united them in their determination to achieve victory'.[83] Logue went through the text, marking pauses between words to make it easier for him to read out. He also changed a few words: 'government', which the King might have stumbled over, was replaced with the easier to pronounce 'ourselves'; while, later in the speech, 'call' took the place of 'summon'.

Logue was struck by the sadness in the King's voice as he read. Logue tried his best to cheer him up, reminding him of how he and the King and Queen had sat in that same room for an hour on coronation night before the broadcast he had made then—which he had approached with equal trepidation. They laughed and reflected on how much had happened in the two and a half years since. At that moment, the door at the other end of the room opened and in came the Queen—looking, as an infatuated Logue put it, 'Royal and lovely'. She was, he thought, as he bowed over her hand, 'the loveliest woman I have ever seen'.

With three minutes to go, it was time to move into the broadcasting room. As they crossed the corridor, the King beckoned to Frederick Ogilvie—who had succeeded Reith as BBC director-general in 1938—to join them. The room had just been redecorated and was bright and cheerful, but the mood was sombre. The King knew just how much was riding on this speech,

210

which would be heard by millions of people across the Empire.

After about fifty seconds, the red light came on. Logue looked at the King and smiled as he stepped up to the microphone. As the clock in the Quadrangle struck six, a smile twitched the corner of his mouth and, with great feeling, he began to speak.

In this grave hour, perhaps the most fateful in our history, I send to every household of my peoples, both at home and overseas, this message, spoken with the same depth of feeling for each one of you as if I were able to cross your threshold and speak to you myself.

For the second time in the lives of most of us we are at war. Over and over again we have tried to find a peaceful way out of the differences between ourselves and those who are now our enemies. But it has been in vain. We have been forced into a conflict. For we are called, with our allies, to meet the challenge of a principle which, if it were to prevail, would be fatal to any civilised order in the world.

It is the principle which permits a state, in the selfish pursuit of power, to disregard its treaties and its solemn pledges; which sanctions the use of force, or threat of force, against the sovereignty and independence of other states. Such a principle, stripped of all disguise, is surely the mere primitive doctrine that might is right; and if this principle were established throughout the world, the freedom of our own country and of the whole British

211

Commonwealth of Nations would be in danger. But far more than this—the peoples of the world would be kept in the bondage of fear, and all hopes of settled peace and of the security of justice and liberty among nations would be ended.

This is the ultimate issue which confronts us. For the sake of all that we ourselves hold dear, and of the world's order and peace, it is unthinkable that we should refuse to meet the challenge.

It is to this high purpose that I now call my people at home and my peoples across the seas, who will make our cause their own. I ask them to stand calm, firm, and united in this time of trial. The task will be hard. There may be dark days ahead, and war can no longer be confined to the battlefield. But we can only do the right as we see the right, and reverently commit our cause to God. If one and all we keep resolutely faithful to it, ready for whatever service or sacrifice it may demand, then, with God's help, we shall prevail.

May He bless and keep us all.

When it was all over and the red light had faded, Logue extended his hand to the King. 'Congratulations on your first wartime speech,' he said. The King, his ordeal behind him, simply stated, 'I expect I will have to do a lot more.' As they walked out of the door, the Queen was waiting in the passage. 'That was good, Bertie,' she said.

The King went to have his photograph taken and Logue stayed with the others in the passage.

'Bertie hardly slept at all last night, he was so worried, but now that we have taken the decisive step he is much more cheerful,' the Queen told him.

Then the King came back and they all said goodbye, and as Logue bowed over the Queen's hand she said, 'I will have to speak to the women. Will you help me with the speech?' Logue told her it would be a great honour.

It was a sign of the importance attached to the speech that the next day's newspapers reported that the King had 'consented' to have 15 million copies of the text printed, with a facsimile of his signature, which would then be sent to every household in the country. This massive mail shot never happened, however: officials estimated that the exercise would require 250 tons of paper, which was already beginning to be in short supply, while the Post Office was alarmed at the extra burden it would impose on its already depleted staff. It was decided that the £35,000 the whole operation would have cost could be better spent elsewhere—not least since the newspapers had printed it in full anyway, accompanied by a photograph of the King dressed for the occasion in his admiral's uniform. As ever, he was portrayed sitting down at the microphone even though, as always, he had been standing up.

In the ensuing days and weeks other cutbacks came into effect. On 25 September petrol rationing was introduced, with people restricted to a mere six gallons a month. London turned almost overnight into a country village. Rationing of food, fuel and other items followed at the beginning of 1940. The Logues were lucky: the woods at the

213

end of the garden provided them with fuel and there was plenty of space to grow fruit and vegetables. Valentine was handy with a gun and often used to bring home rabbits for dinner.

There was also one major source of joy for the Logues: early on 8 September Laurie's wife Jo gave birth to a baby girl, Alexandra. At the time, Tony, who had always done so much to cheer up the place, was preparing to go to university in Leeds where, following in the footsteps of his elder brother, he was to study medicine (his original choice had been London but war changed his plans). With some sadness, his parents saw him on to the train at King's Cross on 5 October. 'His being away takes a lot of laughter out of my life,' wrote Myrtle in her diary.

*   *   *

War or no war, the State Opening of Parliament was due to take place that November—and the King looked to Logue to help him make sure that the speech he had to make went smoothly. There had been some speculation that the King would not appear at all, with details of the government's programme to be read out by the Lord Chancellor.

In the event he turned up in person, but this was to be a State Opening unlike any other. The ceremonial and ornate costumes that were traditionally such an important part of the occasion were abandoned. The King and Queen arrived at the Palace of Westminster by car rather than royal coach and with the minimum of retinue; the King wore a naval uniform; the Queen was in velvet and furs embellished with pearls against the cold. For commentators, the quiet solemnity of the occasion was in sharp contrast to the vulgar fanfare accompanying Hitler's public appearances.

The speech itself, which in peacetime would have set out the government's proposed legislative programme, was short and to the point: 'The prosecution of the war demands the energies of all my subjects,' the King began. Besides telling MPs that they would be asked to make 'further financial provision for the conduct of the war', it gave nothing else away.

The year also brought one last major speech—the Christmas message. With the nation at war, everyone, the King included, knew there could be no question of his not addressing his subjects. It was decided that he would deliver a personal message at the end of the BBC's *Round the Empire* programme on the afternoon of 25 December.

Striking the right tone was a challenge: although the conflict was now well into its fourth month, nothing much had actually happened, as least as far as Britain's civilian population was concerned. The popular perception of a 'phoney war' was at its height. Despite the occasional false alarm, all was quiet on the Western Front and the much-feared air raids had not happened. Many of the children who had been evacuated to the countryside had since returned home. The only real action had been at sea and it was not going well for Britain: on 13 October a skilful U-boat commander managed to penetrate the defences at Scapa Flow, off the north-east coast of Scotland, and sank the battleship *Royal Oak* while she was at anchor, with the loss of more than 830 lives.

British convoys bringing vital supplies across the North Atlantic were harassed by the German navy. A rare success was the destruction of the German 'pocket' battleship the *Graf Spee*, during the Battle of the River Plate, off the coast of Uruguay.

The mood, in short, was one of anticlimax; apathy and complacency were rife—which the King set out to counter. He spoke of what he had seen at first hand: of the Royal Navy, 'upon which, throughout the last four months, had burst the storm of ruthless and unceasing war'; of the Air Force, 'who were daily adding laurels to those that their fathers had won'; and of the British Expeditionary Force in France: 'Their task is hard. They are waiting, and waiting is a trial of nerve and discipline.'

'A new year is at hand,' he continued. 'We cannot tell what it will bring. If it brings peace, how thankful we shall all be. If it brings continued struggle we shall remain undaunted.

'In the meantime, I feel that we may all find a message of encouragement in the lines which, in my closing words, I would like to say to you.'

At that point, apparently at his own initiative, the King quoted some lines from a hitherto unknown poem he had just been sent. It was written by Minnie Louise Haskins who taught at the London School of Economics, and had been privately published in 1908.

'"And I said to the man who stood at the gate of the year: 'Give me a light that I may tread safely into the unknown.' And he replied: 'Go out into the darkness and put your hand into the Hand of God. That shall be to you better than light and safer than a known way.'"'

216

'May that Almighty hand guide and uphold us all.'

The King had dreaded delivering this Christmas message, like almost every other major speech before it. 'This is always an ordeal for me & I don't begin to enjoy Christmas until after it is over,' he wrote in his diary that day.[84] Yet there is no doubting the huge and positive impact that it had on popular morale.

The poem, which Haskins had entitled 'God Knows', also became hugely popular, although under the title 'The Gate of the Year'. It was reproduced on cards and widely published. Its words had a deep impact on the Queen, who had it engraved on brass plaques and was to have it fixed to the gates of the King George VI Memorial Chapel at Windsor Castle, where the King was interred. When she died in 2002, its words were read out at her state funeral.

However successful the King's Christmas message, there was a curious postscript that reflected the continued awareness among members of the public of his speaking problem (coupled with their desire to help him). On 28 December Tommy Lascelles passed on to Logue a letter sent to him from Anthony McCreadie, the rector of John Street Secondary School in Glasgow.

'No one knows that I am writing this note and no one shall ever know I wrote it,' McCreadie began conspiratorially. He went on, without further ado, to explain a technique that the King should employ when making his next broadcast. 'Let him lean on his left elbow and place the back of his hand below his chin—forking his neck between thumb and

217

fingers. Then let him press his chin *firmly* on his hand—exerting a strong pressure up and down when he has difficulty at a sound. This will control his muscles and all difficulty will vanish in the future . . . I humbly hope he will carry out my infallible plan.'

It is not clear if the King was ever passed McCreadie's advice—let alone if he tried to implement it.

CHAPTER THIRTEEN

Dunkirk and the Dark Days

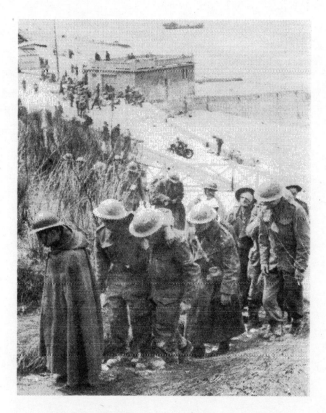

The evacuation from Dunkirk was one of the
Allies' lowest points during World War Two

At one minute to nine on the evening of Friday 24 May 1940, cinemas across Britain shut down their programmes; crowds of people began to gather outside radio shops and a hush fell over clubs and hotel lounges. Millions more were gathered around their radios at home as the King prepared to make his first speech to the nation since his Christmas address at Sandringham. Lasting twelve and a half minutes, it was also to be his longest— and a major test of all the hours he had spent with Logue.

The occasion was Empire Day, which during wartime gained additional resonance from the huge contribution being made by many thousands of people across the Empire to the war against Hitler in Europe. Appropriately, the King's words were to be heard at the end of a programme called *Brothers in Arms*. Featuring men and women born and brought up overseas, the programme, the BBC claimed, would 'demonstrate in no uncertain fashion the unity and strength of which Empire Day is the symbol'.

Britain needed all the help it could get from the Empire. The phoney war had come to a sudden and dramatic end. In April the Nazis had invaded Denmark and Norway. Allied troops landed in Norway in an attempt to defend the country, but by the end of the month the southern areas were in German hands. In early June the Allies evacuated the north and on the ninth Norwegian forces laid down their arms.

The Nazis' successes in Scandinavia brought the long-running pressure on Chamberlain to a head in the so-called Norway debate, during which the former cabinet minister Leo Amery famously quoted to the hapless prime minister the words that Oliver Cromwell had used to the Long Parliament: 'You have sat too long here for any good you have been doing. Depart, I say, and let us have done with you. In the name of God, go.'

Despite the political forces ranged against him, Chamberlain won the vote on 8 May by 281 to 200, but many of his own supporters abstained or voted against him. There was a growing clamour to widen the coalition to include Labour, but that party's MPs refused to serve under Chamberlain. There was speculation that he might be succeeded by Lord Halifax, who had been one of the main architects of appeasement since replacing Eden as foreign secretary in March 1938.

Although Halifax enjoyed the support of both the Conservative Party and the King, and was acceptable to Labour, he realized that there was a better man for the job. When Chamberlain resigned two days later, he was replaced instead by Winston Churchill, who formed a new coalition government including Conservative, Labour and Liberal MPs as well as non-party figures. That same day, German forces marched into Belgium, the Netherlands and Luxembourg.

The Nazis rapidly tightened their grip. At five o'clock in the morning of 13 May, the King was woken to take a call from Queen Wilhelmina of the Netherlands. At first he thought it was a hoax—but not once she began to speak and urgently begged his help in having more aircraft sent to defend her beleaguered country. It was too late; a few hours afterwards the Queen's daughter

Princess Juliana, her German-born husband Prince Bernhard and their two young daughters arrived in England. Later that day, Wilhelmina was on the phone to the King again, this time from Harwich, to which she had travelled aboard a British destroyer after fleeing German attempts to capture her and take her hostage. Her aim was initially to go back and join Dutch forces in Zeeland, in the south-west of the country, which were still resisting, but the military situation had deteriorated so sharply that everyone thought a return was impossible. On 15 May her army capitulated in the face of the German Blitzkrieg. Wilhelmina remained in Buckingham Palace, where she attempted to rally Dutch resistance at a distance.

It was against the background of these dramatic setbacks that Logue was called at 11 a.m. on 21 May by Hardinge and asked to go and see the King at 4 p.m. He arrived fifteen minutes early to find the King's private secretary fretting over yet more bad news from the Continent. German forces, continuing their whirlwind advance across France, had reportedly entered Abbeville, at the mouth of the Somme and fifteen miles from the Channel, cutting the Allied armies in two. The future of the British Expeditionary Force, which had been deployed mainly along the Franco-Belgian border since it had been sent out at the beginning of the war, was looking bleak.

Despite the gravity of the situation, the King appeared in a strangely cheerful mood when Logue was called up to see him. Standing on the balcony, dressed in his military uniform, he was whistling to a young corgi sitting under a plane tree in the garden that was struggling to work out where the sound was coming from. Logue noticed the King's hair was a little greyer on the side of the temples than he remembered it. The strain of war was clearly beginning to take its toll.

They went into a room that was bare of all pictures and valuables save for a vase of flowers. Logue was impressed by the text of the Empire Day speech, which he thought was outstanding and beautifully written, but they nevertheless still went through it together and made some alterations. As they were doing so a second time, there was a light tap at the door. It was the Queen, dressed in powder grey, with a loud diamond butterfly brooch on her left shoulder. While the King was writing out alterations to the text, he talked to Logue about the wonderful efforts the Royal Air Force was making—and 'how proud one should be of the boys from Australia, Canada and New Zealand'. Soon afterwards, Logue went to leave.

'It was a wonderful memory as I said goodbye and bowed over the King's and Queen's hands, the two of them framed in the large window with the sunshine behind them, the King in field marshal uniform and the Queen in grey,' he recalled.

On Empire Day itself, Logue went to the Palace after dinner and, together with the BBC's Wood and Ogilvie, made sure the room had been properly prepared for the broadcast. In case of air raids, Wood had run a cable down into the dugout. 'It didn't matter what happened,' wrote Logue. 'The broadcast would go on.'

The King, dressed in a double-breasted jacket, looked slim and fit. The two of them then went into the broadcasting room which, to Logue's relief, was pleasantly cool: he had left instructions that the windows be left open to prevent a repetition of the previous day's disaster when the unfortunate Queen Wilhelmina had made a lunchtime broadcast to her Dutch colonies in the Caribbean and the room was so hot and stuffy it was practically on fire.

Logue suggested only minor changes to the speech. Rather than beginning 'It is a year ago today', he proposed the King rearrange the text to start instead, 'On Empire Day a year ago'. They had a last run-through of the speech and it took twelve minutes. With just eight minutes to go, the King walked off into his room to practise the emphasis on two or three of the more difficult passages.

A minute before he was due to start speaking, the King walked across the passage into the broadcasting room and stared out of the open window in the failing light. It was a beautiful spring evening and perfectly peaceful. 'It was hard to believe that within a hundred miles of us, men were killing each other,' thought Logue.

The red studio light flashed four times and went dark—the signal to begin. The King took two steps to the table, and Logue squeezed his arm for luck. The gesture spoke volumes about the closeness of the two men's relationship; no one was meant to touch a king unbidden in that way.

'On Empire Day last year I spoke to you, the peoples of the Empire, from Winnipeg, in the heart of Canada,' the King began, adopting the first of Logue's changes. 'We were at peace. On that Empire Day I spoke of the ideals of freedom, justice, and peace upon which our Commonwealth of Free Peoples is founded. The clouds were gathering, but I held fast to the hope that those ideals might yet achieve a fuller and richer development without suffering the grievous onslaught of war. But it was not to be. The evil which we strove unceasingly and with all honesty of purpose to avert fell upon us.'

And so he went on, smiling like a schoolboy (or so Logue thought) whenever he managed a hitherto impossible word without difficulty. The 'decisive struggle' was now upon the people of Britain, the King continued, building up the tension. 'It is no mere territorial conquest that our enemies are seeking; it is the overthrow, complete and final, of this Empire and of everything for which it stands and, after that, the conquest of the world . . .'

There was nothing for Logue to do but just stand and listen, marvelling at the King's voice. When he had spoken his last words, Logue just gripped his hands; both men knew it had been a superb effort.

They didn't dare speak immediately, though; at Logue's insistence, they were trying a new way of working under which the red light—this 'red eye of the little yellow god', as Logue called it—didn't stay on throughout the broadcast. This had the disadvantage of making it difficult to be absolutely certain that they were actually off air. The two men continued to look at each other in silence— 'the King and the commoner and my heart is too full to speak'. The King patted him on the hand.

A few minutes later, Ogilvie came in— 'Congratulations, your Majesty, a wonderful effort', he said—followed by the Queen, kissing

226

her husband and telling him how grand he had been. They all stayed there talking for another five minutes.

'And then,' as Logue put it, 'the King of England says "I want my dinner"—and they all said good night and went down the stairs into another world.'

The King was suitably proud of his effort, and relieved that, despite the fluidity of the military situation, he had not been obliged to make major last-minute changes to the text. 'I was fearful that something might happen to make me have to alter it,' he wrote in his diary that evening. 'I was very pleased with the way I delivered it, & it was easily my best effort. How I hate broadcasting.'[85]

The next morning, the newspapers were full of praise for the speech. The *Daily Telegraph* called it 'a vigorous and inspiring broadcast', adding, 'Reports last night indicated that every word was heard with perfect clarity throughout the United States and in distant parts of the Empire.' Logue's telephone, meanwhile, had been ringing off the hook. 'Everyone is thrilled over The King's Speech,' he wrote in his diary. 'Eric Mieville rang me from Buckingham Palace and told me that the reception all over the world had been tremendous. Whilst we were speaking the King rang for him, so I sent my congratulations through again.' The reaction from the Empire and beyond had also been enthusiastic.

The next day, a Saturday, Logue and Myrtle celebrated the King's success by going to see a matinee of *My Little Chickadee*, a comedy set in the Old West of the 1880s, starring Mae West and W. C. Fields. Afterwards, Valentine took his parents to dinner at a restaurant Myrtle called 'the

Hungarian'. It was the first time they had been there since the war had started, and the band played all Myrtle's favourites.

It would take more than one speech, however fine, to turn the tide of a war which was going against the Allies. Next to fall to the Germans was Belgium. King Léopold III, who was commander-in-chief of his country's forces, had hoped to fight on in support of the Allied course, imitating the heroic example of his father, King Albert, during the First World War. Yet the situation this time was different, and on 25 May, convinced that further resistance was hopeless, Léopold surrendered. Controversially he chose to stay with his people rather than accompany his ministers to France where they attempted to continue to operate as a government-in-exile. However unfairly, he was vilified in Britain as a result. His behaviour during the war divided his own country and sowed the seeds for his abdication just over a decade later.

The British fury at Léopold's capitulation was due in large part to the damaging effect it had on the Allied Forces, whose left flank was now entirely exposed and who now had to fall back to the Channel coast. The only solution was to mount a rescue—and what was to be one of the most dramatic episodes of the war. On 27 May the first of a flotilla of around 700 merchant marine boats, fishing boats, pleasure craft and Royal National Lifeboats began to evacuate British and French troops from the beaches of Dunkirk. By the ninth day, a total of 338,226 soldiers (198,229 British and 139,997 French) had been rescued.

On 4 June, the final day of the evacuation,

Churchill made one of the most memorable speeches of the war—or, indeed, of all time. 'Even though large tracts of Europe and many old and famous States have fallen or may fall into the grip of the Gestapo and all the odious apparatus of Nazi rule, we shall not flag or fail,' he told the House of Commons, going on famously to vow to 'fight on the beaches'.

In her diary the next day, Myrtle noted simply: 'All our men off. God be praised. Have met some of the nurses, they have a story to tell which will live forever.' There were some more immediate worries too: on 1 June, in the midst of the evacuation, she heard that Laurie, their eldest son, had joined the army. Already into his thirties, and with a wife and baby, he was not among the first to be called. At the end of March he received his call-up papers and when Myrtle heard the news, she and Jo had 'a little weep'.

*   *   *

For many ordinary people, what became known as the Dunkirk spirit perfectly described the tendency of Britons to pull together at times of national emergency and adversity. Yet, however great the heroism and however remarkable some of the escapes, there was no disguising the fact that this was no victory. In private, Churchill told his junior ministers that Dunkirk was 'the greatest British military defeat for many centuries'.

The bad news kept on coming. On 14 June Paris was occupied by the German Wehrmacht and then, three days later, Marshal Philippe Pétain (appointed head of state with extraordinary powers) announced that France would ask Germany for an armistice. 'This is the blackest day we have ever known,' wrote Myrtle in her war diary. She heard news of Pétain's announcement from a disgusted bus driver who 'proclaimed to the entire world what he would do to the entire French nation . . . Surely now, there is nobody left who can rat on us. We are all really alone, and if our government gives up there will be a revolution, and I am in it.'

Things were about to get even blacker. Late in the afternoon of 7 September, 364 German bombers, escorted by a further 515 aircraft, carried out air raids on London, with another 133 attacking that night. Their target was the Port of London, but many of the bombs fell on residential areas, killing 436 Londoners and injuring more than 1,600. The Blitz had begun. For the next seventy-five consecutive nights, the bombers targeted London repeatedly. Other important military and industrial centres such as Birmingham, Bristol, Liverpool and Manchester were also hit. By May the following year, when the campaign ended, more than 43,000 civilians, half of them in the capital, had been killed and more than a million homes damaged or destroyed in the London area alone.

Buckingham Palace was also hit several times that September during a daring daylight raid, when both the King and Queen were working there. The bombs caused considerable damage to the Royal Chapel and the inner quadrangle—prompting the Queen famously to declare, 'I'm glad we've been bombed. It makes me feel I can look the East End in the face.' Logue wrote to the King to express his

230

'thankfulness and gratitude to the Most High' at his narrow escape from what he called 'a dastardly attempt on your life'. He added, 'It did not seem possible that even the Germans would descend to such depths of infamy.'

Tommy Lascelles wrote back to Logue four days later to thank him for his expression of concern, which the King and Queen had greatly appreciated. 'T.M. [their majesties] are none the worse for their experience,' he added. 'I hope you manage to get some sleep now and then.'

In the weeks that followed, Logue and the King kept up an occasional correspondence. The monarch was often surprisingly frank about his feelings, such as after he visited Coventry on 15 November in the immediate aftermath of a devastating overnight raid on the city. More than 500 tons of high explosive bombs and incendiaries were dropped, turning the centre into a sea of flames and killing nearly 600 people. The cathedral was almost completely destroyed and the King spent hours tramping through the rubble. The effect of his visit on the city's morale was huge, although the King himself was overwhelmed by the sheer scale of destruction. 'What could I say to these poor people who had lost everything, sometimes their families[;] words were inadequate,' he asked Logue.

Amid the stress and misery there were some lighter moments. A few days later, when the King was practising his speech for that year's State Opening of Parliament, he greeted Logue grinning like a schoolboy. 'Logue, I've got the jitters,' he declared. 'I woke up at one o'clock after dreaming I was in parliament with my mouth wide open and couldn't say a word.' Although both men laughed heartily, it brought home to Logue that even now, after all the years they had spent working together, the King's speech impediment still weighed heavily on him.

Logue was invited back to Windsor on Christmas Eve, and then again on Christmas Day, to help with the speech. This year, as the previous one, there could be no question of the King not addressing the Empire.

The weather was cold but cheerful. Logue felt he couldn't chance the trains and so took the Green Line bus to Windsor instead. 'I had been standing in the cold all night and when the door was opened, and we got in, the cold hit you,' he wrote. 'It was like getting into an Ice House. I got colder and colder and when I reached Windsor, I fell out of the bus a frozen mass.' The walk up to the castle thawed him a little; a glass of sherry with Mieville after he arrived helped further, as did the coal fire burning in the grate. He was also delighted by a gold cigarette case given to him by the Queen.

After a Christmas dinner of boar's head and prunes, Logue followed the King to his study and they got down to work. Logue did not like the speech; as far as he was concerned there was nothing for the King to get his teeth into, but there was little he could do about it. In it, the King warned his people that the future would be hard 'but our feet are planted on the path of victory and, with the help of God, we shall make our way to justice and to peace'.

*　　　*　　　*

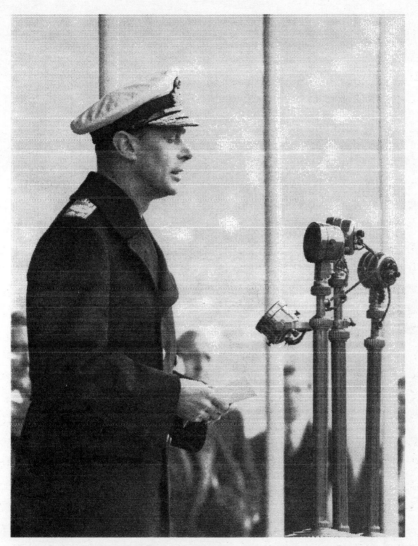

One of George VI's first broadcasts as King in 1937

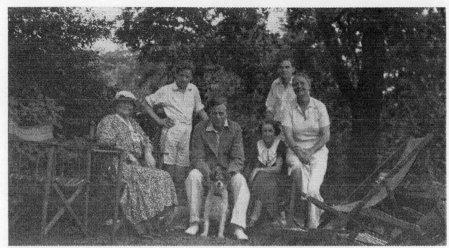

The Logue family relaxing by the tennis courts at Beechgrove, Sydenham Hill *From left: unidentified guest, Antony, Lionel, unidentified guest, Valentine, Myrtle*

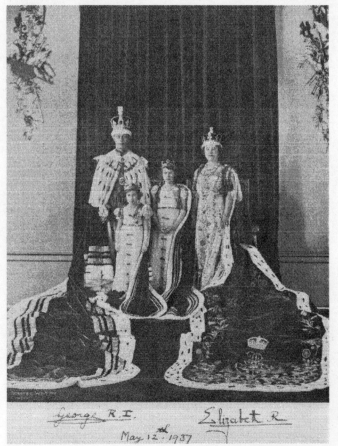

George R.I.
May 12ᵗʰ 1937
Elizabeth R

The Royal Family in Coronation robes. King George VI and Queen Elizabeth with their daughters Princess Elizabeth and Princess Margaret. The King gave Lionel this framed portrait as a gift

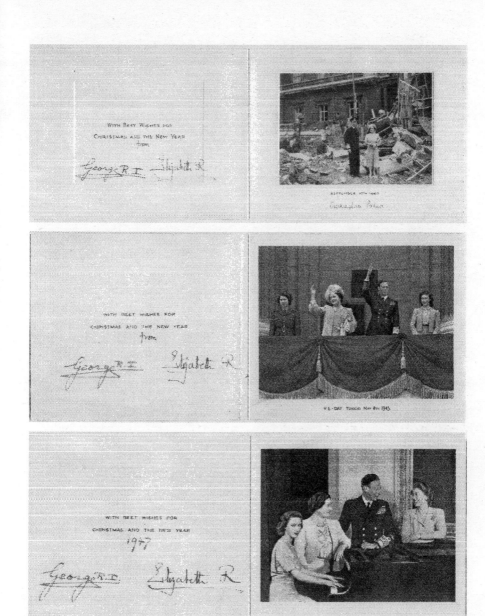

A selection of Christmas cards from the Royal Family. The Logues would continue to receive a card every year until the King's death

BUCKINGHAM PALACE

In this grave hour, perhaps the most fateful in
our history, I send to every household of my peoples,
both at home and overseas, this message, spoken with the
same depth of feeling for each one of you as if I were
able to cross your threshold and speak to you myself.

For the second time in the lives of most of us
we are at war. Over and over again we have tried to find
a peaceful way out of the differences between my
Government and those who are now our enemies. But it
has been in vain. We have been forced into a conflict.
For we are called, with our allies, to meet the challenge
of a principle which, if it were to prevail, would be
fatal to any civilized order in the world.

It is the principle which permits a State, in the

The speech broadcast on the outbreak of war on
3 September 1939. This is the actual speech from
which the King read, annotated by Lionel to
indicate the pauses the King should make, as well
as highlighting any potentially tricky words

the selfish pursuit of power, to disregard its treaties and
its solemn pledges; which sanctions the use of force, or
the threat of force, against the Sovereignty and independence
of other States.   Such a principle, stripped of all disguise,
is surely the mere primitive doctrine that might is right.
If it were established throughout the world, the freedom of
our own country and of the whole British Commonwealth of
nations would be in danger.   But far more than this - the
peoples of the world would be kept in the bondage of fear,
and all hopes of settled peace and of the security of justice
and liberty among nations would be ended.

This is the ultimate issue which confronts us.   For
the sake of all that we ourselves hold dear, and of the
world's order and peace, it is unthinkable that we should
refuse to meet the challenge.

It is to this high purpose that I now summon my people
at home and my peoples across the Seas, who will make our
cause their own.   I ask them to stand calm, firm and united
in this time of trial.   The task will be hard.   There may be

dark days ahead, and war can no longer be confined to
the battlefield.   But we can only do the right as we
see the right, and reverently commit our cause to God.
If one and all we keep resolutely faithful to it, ready
for whatever service or sacrifice it may demand, then
with God's help, we shall prevail.

May He bless and keep us all.

BUCKINGHAM PALACE

December 16th 1951

My dear Logue,

I am so sorry to hear that you have not been well again though I understand you do still see patients. Thank you so much for sending me the books for my birthday which are most acceptable.

As for myself I have spent a wretched year, culminating in that very severe operation, from which I seem to be making a remarkable recovery. The latter fact is in many ways entirely due to you. Before the operation Price Thomas the surgeon asked to see me breathe. When he saw the diaphragm moving up & down naturally he asked me whether I had always

BUCKINGHAM PALACE

breathed in that way. I said No, I had been taught to breathe like that in 1926 & had gone on doing so. Another feather in your cap you see!! All the exercises I have done since the operation have come very easily due to right breathing. I find no trouble in walking upstairs & there is no extra exertion.

Though with one lung, the right one, the left side ribs still work as well as before & I see no reason why they should not continue to do so.

My voice unfortunately is quite another matter. Due to the infection, & gas & Bronchoscopy & the operation one of the vocal chords is still in a state of paralysis. The voice is getting stronger all the time able but is hardly,

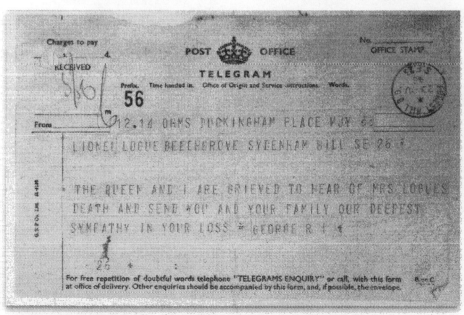

A selection of letters from the King to Lionel, showing his friendly concern for his health, along with the telegram he sent after Myrtle's death

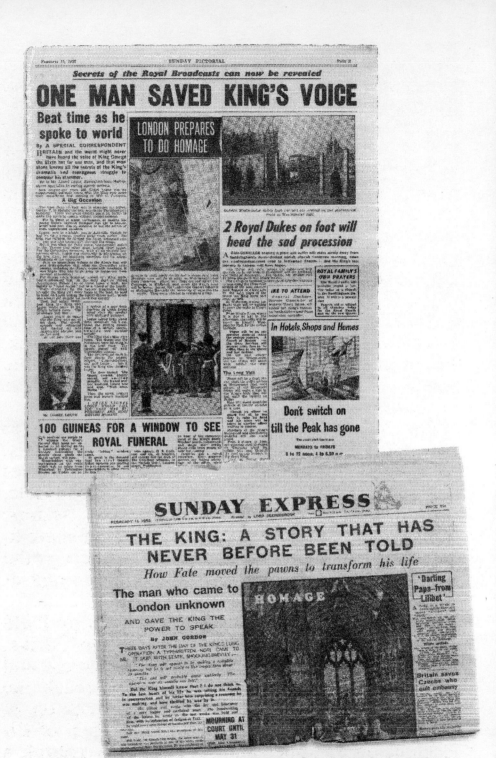

After the King's death in February 1952, the newspapers gave a dramatic spin to the story of his relationship with Lionel

And so it went on. On 22 June 1941 Germany, along with other European Axis members and Finland, invaded the Soviet Union in Operation Barbarossa. The aim was to eliminate the country and communism, providing not just *Lebensraum* but also access to the strategic resources Germany needed to defeat its remaining rivals. In the months that followed, Hitler and his allies made significant gains in Ukraine and the Baltic region, as well as laying siege to Leningrad and coming close to the outskirts of Moscow. Yet Hitler had failed to attain his objective and Stalin retained a considerable part of his military potential. On 5 December the Russians began a counter-attack. Two days later the Japanese attacked the American fleet at Pearl Harbor, bringing in the might of the United States on the Allied side.

The Axis powers continued to make advances through 1942: Japanese forces swept through Asia, conquering Burma, Malaya, the Dutch East Indies and the Philippines. The Germans, meanwhile, ravaged Allied shipping off America's Atlantic coast, and in June launched a summer offensive to seize the oilfields of the Caucasus and occupy the Kuban steppe. The Soviets made their stand at Stalingrad.

War was also raging in Africa, where Field Marshal Erwin Rommel's Panzerarmee Afrika, composed of German and Italian infantry and mechanized units, was threatening to reach the gates of Cairo. Rommel opened his attack on 26 May, forced the evacuation by the French of Bir Hachim on 11 June and laid siege to Tobruk a week later. He then swept eastwards out of Libya

233

into Egypt, reaching El Alamein, sixty miles west of Alexandria, on 1 July. It was a bitter blow to the Allies: Churchill, in Washington, flew back to face a censure motion in the Commons, which he won easily.

Then came the turning point in Africa and, it could be argued, the war. The British forces counter-attacked, repulsing Rommel. The Germans dug in, however, and a stalemate ensued, during which Lieutenant-General Bernard Montgomery was appointed commander of the Eighth Army. On 23 October the Allies attacked again, with Montgomery's 200,000 men and 1,100 tanks ranged against the Axis's 115,000 men and 559 tanks: Rommel was back home in Germany on sick leave, but hurried back to lead his men. The numbers were overwhelmingly against him and on 2 November he warned Hitler his forces were not capable of offering any more effective opposition. The Nazi leader would not tolerate any talk of surrender: 'It would not be the first time in history that a strong will has triumphed over the bigger battalions,' Hitler replied the next day. 'As to your troops, you can show them no other road than that to victory or death.'

Logue was one of the first to hear of Montgomery's victory. On the afternoon of 4 November he was at the Palace with the King, going through a speech he was due to give at the State Opening of Parliament, set for the twelfth, when the telephone rang. The King had given orders that he was not to be disturbed unless he was wanted urgently. With a quizzical look, he walked over and picked up the receiver.

The King immediately became excited. 'Yes!

Yes! Well read it out, read it out,' he said, before adding, 'The enemy is in full retreat. Good news, thanks,' and hung up. Smiling, he turned to Logue. "Did you hear that?' he asked, and repeated the gist of the news. 'Well,' he said. 'That's grand.'

That evening the King wrote in his diary: 'A victory at last, how good it is for the nerves.'[86] Four days later, Allied forces landed in Morocco and Algeria, both nominally in the hands of the Vichy France regime. Operation Torch, intended to open a second front in North Africa, was under way.

*   *   *

Amid such drama, yet another Christmas speech was looming. A couple of days before, Logue rehearsed it with the King, whom he had found in excellent form. The speech itself required a little surgery; Logue wasn't keen on passages that Churchill had written into the text as they just didn't seem right coming out of the King's mouth. 'It was typical Churchill and could have been recognised by anyone,' Logue complained in his diary. 'With the King's help, we cut out adjectives and the Prime Minister.'

The weather that year was lovely, despite a touch of fog, and there was no repeat of the snow of the previous two years. Logue was again summoned to join the royal family for the festivities. He thought the Christmas tree looked much nicer and better decorated than the year before; a decoration Myrtle had sent had made all the difference. When the Queen came in, she walked over to Logue and told him how pleased she was to see him. To his surprise, she then asked him to repeat a trick he had been showing a couple of the equerries before lunch: how to breathe using only one lung. He happily did so, but warned her and the two princesses not to attempt the trick themselves.

Just after 2.30, Logue followed the King into his study to go through the speech for one last time. At 2.55 they entered the broadcasting room, he and Wood synchronized watches and at 2.58 the Queen came in to wish her husband good luck. A few seconds later the three red lights went on and, with a glance in Logue's direction, the King began.

'It is at Christmas more than any other time, that we are conscious of the dark shadow of war,' he started. 'Our Christmas festival today must lack many of the happy, familiar features that it has had from our childhood . . . But though its outward observances may be limited, the message of Christmas remains eternal and unchanged. It is a message of thankfulness and of hope—of thankfulness to the Almighty for His great mercies, of hope for the return to this earth of peace and good will.' Logue followed the printed text for a couple of paragraphs, but then gave up— he realized there was no need to do so any more.

During the speech, the King spoke of the great contribution being made to the war effort by the other members of the Empire—and also by the Americans. He ended with a story once told by Abraham Lincoln about a boy who was carrying a much smaller child up a hill. 'Asked whether the heavy burden was not too much for him, the boy answered, "It's not a burden, it's my brother."'

After exactly twelve minutes it was all over and

Logue was delighted by what he had heard. 'It is a grand thing to be the first to congratulate a King, and letting a few seconds go by to make sure we were off the air, I grabbed him by the arm, and in my excitement said "splendid",' Logue wrote in his diary. 'He grinned and said, "I think that's the best we have done, Logue. I will be back in London in February, let us keep the lessons going." The Queen came in, kissed him fondly and said, "That was splendid, Bertie".'

The newspapers were full of praise for the royal performance. 'Both in manner and in matter, the King's broadcast yesterday was the most mature and inspiriting that he has yet made,' commented the *Glasgow Herald*. 'It worthily maintained the tradition of Christmas Day broadcasts.' Churchill, the greatest orator of them all, rang to congratulate him on how well he had done.

On Boxing Day the King sent Logue a handwritten letter that reflected quite how pleased he had been with how it had gone.

My dear Logue,
I'm so glad that my broadcast went off so well yesterday. I felt altogether different and I had no fear of the microphone. I am sure that those visits that you have paid me have done me a great deal of good and I must keep them up during the new year.
Thank you so very much for all your help.
With all good wishes for 1943
I am
Yours very sincerely
George R.I.

Logue wrote back full of enthusiasm. 'Today, my telephone has been beating a "tattoo", all manner of people have been ringing to congratulate you, saying how they wished they could write and let you know how much they enjoyed the broadcast,' he said. He singled out for praise the way the King had approached the dreaded microphone 'almost as if it were your friend' and how he had never looked as if he were being held up.

CHAPTER FOURTEEN

The Tide Turns

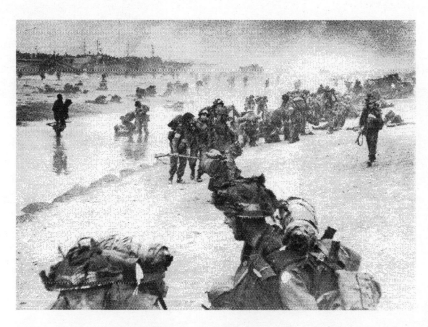

On 6 June 1944 the Allies finally returned to
mainland Europe

By the summer of 1943, after two years of unremitting bad news, the war was beginning to go the Allies' way. The battle for North Africa had ended in triumph. Then, on 10 July, the British Eighth Army, under General Bernard Montgomery, and the US Seventh Army, under General George Patton, began their combined assault on Sicily, which was to serve as the springboard for an invasion of the Italian mainland. A fortnight later Mussolini was deposed, and on 3 September the government of Pietro Badoglio agreed to unconditional surrender; the following month, Italy declared war on Germany.

There were other causes for celebration elsewhere: the much-feared *Tirpitz*, the largest battleship ever built in Europe, was badly damaged in September 1943 by a daring raid by British midget submarines while she was at anchor. Then, on Boxing Day, the battle cruiser *Scharnhorst* was sunk off Norway's North Cape. The battle of the Atlantic had effectively been won by the Allies. There was good news from the Far East, too: the Japanese advances were being stemmed, and the British and Americans were preparing to fight back.

Yet the war still had some time to run. The Germans were putting up fierce resistance both in Italy and on the Russian front, while the Japanese were a long way from being defeated. Churchill, over-optimistically, told the King he thought the Germans might well be beaten before the end of 1944, but feared it might take until 1946 to secure

241

victory in the Far East.

The King was keen to take advantage of the improving situation to visit his victorious armies in the field and congratulate them on their achievements. He had made such a trip before, in December 1939, when he visited the British Expeditionary Force in France, but the situation had deteriorated so badly in the meantime that there had been no thought of a repetition. In June 1943, however—travelling incognito as 'General Lyon' for security reasons—he set off on a far more ambitious two-week trip to North Africa, during which he inspected British and American forces in Algeria and Libya. On his way back, he also made a brief visit to the 'island fortress' of Malta whose highly strategic position in the Mediterranean had earned it a battering from the Germans. Everywhere he went, he received a predictably enthusiastic reception.

Logue, by contrast, was living the ebb and flow of the Allied forces' fortunes vicariously through the experiences of his sons. Laurie had been first to be called up, in 1940, and was serving in the Royal Army Services Corps. Thanks to the experience of the catering industry he had acquired while working at Lyons, he was put in the branch of the corps responsible for transporting food. He was sent to Africa, where he served in the 'Gideon Force' under the eccentric Colonel Orde Wingate, which in May 1941 helped drive the Italians out of Ethiopia and restored Haile Selassie to the throne. In February 1942 he was promoted to second lieutenant and, a month later, was mentioned in dispatches. By June, he had made lieutenant.

Next to be called up was Tony. After just a year of medicine at Leeds University, he joined the Scots Guards in 1941 and, following a spell at Sandhurst, went to North Africa. Valentine, meanwhile, was pursuing his medical career on the home front: after a spell in general surgery, dealing with the victims of the Blitz, he switched in 1941 to the demanding and rapidly developing field of neuro-surgery. He was sent first to a hospital in St Albans, where he specialized in head injuries, and then on to Edinburgh.

Logue, himself, now aged in his sixties, was too old to serve in the forces, but he did work three nights a week as an air-raid warden. His health was beginning to suffer: in August 1943 he went into hospital to have an operation on a stomach ulcer. The King, who was having his traditional summer break at Balmoral, was kept informed of Logue's progress by Mieville, who also arranged for him to spend some time by the sea to convalesce. On 23 October Logue wrote to the King: 'I rejoice to say that I am quite recovered, and I am looking forward to attending on you on your return. It has been a long three months. As it is the first ulcer I have ever had, I did not take to it too kindly, but I thank the Good Lord that everything has been a great success.'

The war brought financial as well as medical problems: the young men who made up the overwhelming bulk of Logue's patients had, like his own sons, been called up into the armed forces. The constant aerial bombardment during the Blitz also dissuaded others from making the trip to London for a consultation. For that reason, a gift of £500 that the King sent him in January 1941—'a

243

personal present from His Majesty in recognition of the very valuable personal services you have rendered'—was especially welcome.

'That you with all your great responsibility and worry should thank me and help me so naturally has overwhelmed me,' a grateful Logue wrote back. 'My humble service has always been at your disposal, and it has been the great privilege of my life to serve you . . . Your kindly thoughtfulness has touched me many times, and my sincere and heartfelt wish is that I may be spared to serve you for many years.'

One-off gifts, however welcome, were not enough to solve the Logues' financial problems. Their big house on Sydenham Hill was also turning into something of a burden. 'Beechgrove has been terribly hard to keep going, as there is no labour,' Logue complained in a letter to Myrtle's younger brother Rupert in June 1942. 'Myrtle has no servants at all, and we cannot even get a man to help cut the lawns, so a house with 25 rooms, and 5 bathrooms these times is a bit of an incubus, and as I am not allowed to use the motor mower but have to use the heavy old "push" one, I would not like to say how big the corns on my hands [are].' So they got a sheep to keep the lawn down instead.

Logue's work with the King did not bring just financial rewards: on the eve of the coronation he had been made a member of the Royal Victorian Order; in the Birthday Honours List of June 1943 he was promoted to the rank of commander. The investiture was held on 4 July the following year. He was also honoured to be appointed as the British Society of Speech Therapists' representative on the board of the British Medical

Association—although, as he wrote to Rupert, 'I only wish these things had come 20 years ago, when one could enjoy them so much more. I am 62 and find I cannot do the things I once could.'

There were expressions of gratitude, too, from some of the patients, letters from whom are included among Logue's papers. A fifty-three-year-old civil servant named C. B. Archer, from Wimbledon, south-west London, wrote on 30 November 1943 to thank Logue for completely curing him of the stammer from which he had been suffering since the age of eight, apparently through teaching him to breathe abdominally. 'It was a lucky day for me a little over six months ago when I first got into touch with you,' Archer wrote. 'I think only a stammerer can really appreciate what a different world I live in now. It is as if a load has been lifted from my mind.' The man's letter, running to five hand-written pages, gave an insight into the blight that the stammer had cast over his professional as well as his private life.

'My stammering has been a terrific drawback to me in the civil service,' he continued. 'Otherwise I should probably have been an assistant secretary by now. All promotions are as a result of interviews by a Promotion Board and you imagine what a sorry show I made in front of them.'

The following month, Logue received an especially effusive letter from a Tom Mallin, in Sutton Coldfield, Birmingham, noting how both his mother and his friends had noticed the difference since he had started consulting Logue. 'My friends all say I have "changed"—yes—but for the better,' Mallin wrote. 'Now I begin to realise that the voice can be so beautiful, satisfying and

245

expressive, it is a wonder I haven't tumbled to it before . . . Sir, how can I ever thank you for making me happy?' He was due to go to an interview a couple of weeks later, 'and I will remember everything you have taught me. I will be sure of impressing them'.[87]

*　　　*　　　*

The war, in the meantime, was moving towards another of its decisive turning points. On Thursday 1 June 1944, at 9.30 p.m., Logue received a call from Lascelles, who had been promoted to the King's private secretary after the rather abrasive Hardinge had been effectively forced out in July 1943. 'My master wants to know if you can come to Windsor tomorrow, Friday, for lunch,' he asked. Logue was happy to oblige.

Logue took the 12.44 train. Lascelles, whom he met in the equerries' room, was in a very serious mood. 'Sorry I cannot tell you much about the broadcast,' he said. 'It is, as a matter of fact, a call to prayer, and takes about five minutes, and strange as it may seem, I cannot tell you when it is, as you have probably guessed that it is to be given on the night of D-Day, at nine o'clock.'

Logue went off to have lunch with the equerries, the ladies-in-waiting and the captain of the guard, and afterwards, the King sent for him. He was in his study with the blinds drawn down—but the room was still extremely hot. He looked tired and weary and told Logue he wasn't sleeping very well. But when they went through the speech, Logue was charmed by it. He timed it: five and a half minutes precisely.

246

Lascelles had not had to explain what he meant by D-Day. The military terminology for the day chosen for the Allied assault on Europe had long since passed into common parlance. But when— and where—that assault would take place remained a closely guarded secret. The element of surprise was essential if the Allies were to succeed, and they had gone to extraordinary and ingenious lengths to feed disinformation to the Germans.

It had been seventeen months earlier, at the Casablanca Conference in January 1943, that Roosevelt and Churchill had agreed on a full-scale invasion of Nazi-occupied Europe using a combination of British and American forces. Churchill, who was keen to avoid a repetition of the costly frontal assaults of the First World War, had proposed invading the Balkans, with the aim of linking up with Soviet forces and then possibly bringing in Turkey on the side of the Allies. The Americans preferred an invasion of Western Europe, however—and their view prevailed. The decision was confirmed at the Quebec conference of August 1943. The operation was named Operation Overlord, and by that winter the choice of landing point had been narrowed down to either the Pas-de-Calais area or Normandy. On Christmas Eve, General Eisenhower was appointed Supreme Commander of the Allied Expeditionary Force (SCAEF).

Plans for the operation were outlined by Eisenhower and his commanders at a meeting held on 15 May in a classroom of St Paul's School—the unusual venue was chosen apparently because General Montgomery, commander of the 21st Army Group, to which all of the invasion ground

247

forces belonged, had been educated there. In the days that followed, more and more forces were concentrated in southern England; the invasion was imminent.

D-Day was initially tentatively set for 5 June, but the weather that weekend was poor: it was cold and wet and there was a gale blowing from the west and high seas, all of which would make it impossible to launch landing craft from larger ships at sea. Low cloud, meanwhile, would prevent Allied aircraft from finding their targets. The operation required a day close to full moon; one was due on that Monday. Delaying for nearly a month and sending the troops back to their embarkation camps would be a huge and difficult operation and so, advised by his chief meteorologist of a brief clear improvement in the weather the next day, Eisenhower took the momentous decision of going for 6 June.

Hours later, Operation Neptune—the name given to the first, assault phase of Operation Overlord—began: shortly after midnight, 24,000 British, American, Canadian and Free French airborne troops landed. Then, starting at 6.30 a.m. British Double Summer Time, the first Allied infantry and armoured divisions embarked along a fifty-mile stretch of the Normandy coast. By the end of the day, more than 165,000 troops had come ashore; over 5,000 ships were involved. It was the largest amphibious invasion of all time.

That evening at six o'clock, Logue arrived, as arranged, at the Palace; he was shown in to see the King fifteen minutes later. The speech was scheduled for nine o'clock and the atmosphere was tense. But there were also some comic moments:

just as Logue was taking the King through his voice exercises, they caught sight out of the window of a procession of five people in the garden of Buckingham Palace, among them a policeman. As they watched, the woman put a net over her head, which made Logue think they were trying to coax a swarm of bees into a box. 'The King got quite excited, and wanted to go out and give them a hand,' observed Logue. 'It only wanted me to say yes, and he would have opened the window and gone on to the lawn—but it wouldn't do to have the King chance being stung by a bee just before a broadcast, so curious as I was I had to pretend that I was not interested.'

After trying the speech through once, they went downstairs to the air-raid shelter. Logue was fascinated by it. 'What a beautiful place,' he wrote. 'It would do me as a residence—full of peculiar furniture and the latest ideas for heating and light.' Wood of the BBC was also there. They ran through the text; it went well: the speech ran to five and a half minutes, and they needed to make just two alterations. The only problem was the loud ticking of a clock, coming from the King's bedroom, which had to be silenced for fear of it spoiling the broadcast.

After they had finished, they returned to the King's room—and he went immediately back to the windows to see what had become of the bees. The people had all gone, leaving behind a small box. As Logue was sitting making small changes to the speech, the Queen came in, and to his amusement, the King 'explained like a schoolboy, what had happened about the bees, even going down on his knees to explain the detail of the capture'. The Queen also became excited, and said, 'Oh Bertie, I wish I had been here.'

That evening, as Britons gathered around their radios, the King spoke:

> Four years ago our nation and Empire stood alone against an overwhelming enemy with our backs to the wall, tested as never before in our history, and we survived that test. The spirit of the people, resolute and dedicated, burned like a bright flame, surely, from those unseen fires which nothing can quench.
>
> Once more the supreme test has to be faced. This time the challenge is not to fight to survive, but to fight to win the final victory for the good cause. Once again, what is demanded from us all is something more than courage, more than endurance.

The King went on to call for a 'revival of the spirit, a new unconquerable reserve' and to 'renew that crusading impulse on which we entered the war and met its darkest hour'. He concluded with a quote from verse 11 of Psalm 29: 'The Lord will give strength unto his people; the Lord will bless his people with peace.'

The speech perfectly fitted the national mood. While the front pages of the newspapers the following morning carried graphic accounts of the landings, the leader writers reacted with pride at what was seen as a chance for Britain finally to reverse the indignity it had suffered four years earlier at Dunkirk. The King received a number of letters of gratitude that touched him deeply—none more than the one sent by his mother, Queen

Mary. 'I am glad you liked my broadcast,' he wrote in reply. 'It was a great opportunity to call everybody to prayer. I have wanted to do it for a long time.'[88]

*   *   *

Operation Overlord proved a success. The battle for Normandy continued for more than two months. On 21 August, after a battle that raged for more than a week, the so-called 'Falaise Pocket' was closed, trapping 50,000 German troops inside. Days later, Paris was liberated—the German garrison occupying the city surrendered on 25 August—and by the thirtieth the last German troops had retreated across the River Seine. Brussels was liberated by British forces on 3 September. By October, German forces had been almost completely driven from France and Belgium and from the southern portion of the Netherlands.

The Allies were also moving forward in Italy, with their aim the capture of Rome. During the early morning hours of 22 January 1944, troops of the Fifth Army had swarmed ashore on a fifteen-mile stretch of Italian beach near the pre-war resort towns of Anzio and Nettuno, taking the Germans almost completely by surprise. The initial landings were carried out so flawlessly and the resistance so light that British and American units had gained their first day's objectives by noon, and moved three to four miles inland by nightfall. The British forces included the Scots Guards, among whom was Second Lieutenant Antony Logue—Lionel's youngest.

In a classic military blunder, however, Major General John Lucas, the commander of the US VI Corps, then threw away any element of surprise by delaying his advance in order to consolidate his beachhead. When he did try and move forward at the end of the month, he faced fierce resistance from the Germans under General Albert Kesselring, who in the meantime had had time to move in his reinforcements. These then formed a ring around the beachhead and rained down fire on the Allied troops in the swamp below. Many British lives were lost. By 18 and 19 February things were going so badly for the Allies that it looked as if all might end in another Dunkirk. Miraculously, they survived, but only after a ferocious battle—as a letter from Tony home to his parents, dated Midnight 19 February, and written by torchlight, revealed:

You can tell Val that, until last night I had not taken off my boots or my coat, or removed a stitch of my clothing for 19 days, a very different figure to the debonair figure of peacetime,' he wrote. 'Still, it has been a classic show and one that I feel should live in history forever. I am very proud to have been here and to have participated in my tiny way. The fellows have fought as only the Brigade of Guards can, more than that I cannot say.

For the next two months or so the situation remained static, and then, finally, on 4 June, two days before D-Day, they entered Rome. Tony, who had been promoted the previous month to captain, described the scene in a letter home on 15 June.

I was in a jeep on the second night, one of the most beautiful cities I have ever seen. All was completely quiet and orderly, people enjoying their ordinary lives without disturbance and except for the stream of convoys, no soldiers to be seen, it was the finest occupation I have experienced.

We were in a wood north of Rome when we heard of the second front, and since then we have not stopped. I have had enough ecstatic welcomes over the last fortnight to last me all my days. These northern Italian cities, amongst the most beautiful in the world, have welcomed us right royally, and in most cases the German's fires have not yet gone cold.

Although the momentum across Europe was now clearly with the Allies, Hitler made a last desperate attempt to turn the tide. On 16 December 1944, the German army launched a massive counter-offensive in the Ardennes with the aim of splitting the Western Allies, encircling large portions of their troops and capturing Antwerp, the primary port from which they were supplied.

For those, such as Logue, back in Britain, the days after D-Day also saw the deployment by Hitler of his first secret weapon, the V-1, pilotless planes filled with explosives that were to rain down on London and other cities day and night for much of the next nine months. The effect on morale was severe. 'There is something very inhuman about death-dealing missiles being launched in such an indiscriminate manner,' the Queen wrote to

Queen Mary.[89] There was worse to come: that September the V-1s were followed by the even more terrifying V-2s, ballistic missiles launched from installations in the Netherlands and the Pas de Calais, which fell with no warning on London and the south-east. The first one hit Chiswick, in the west of the capital, on 8 September.

* * *

Despite all the progress he had made over the years with Logue, the King was still far from being a perfect public speaker—as is clearly audible to anyone listening to the recordings of those of his speeches that have survived in the archives. A contemporary analysis was provided in an unsolicited letter that was sent to Lascelles that June. It was written by the Reverend Robert Hyde, the founder of the Boys' Welfare Association, the organization of which the King had become patron more than two decades earlier when he was the Duke of York. Over the years, Hyde had had plenty of opportunities to listen to the King at close quarters and was apparently keen to share his impressions—although he didn't offer any solutions. The letter was nevertheless passed to Logue.

'As you know, I have studied the King's speech for some years, so send you this note for what it is worth,' Hyde wrote. The hesitations, he said, seemed quite consistent. 'Apart from a slight lapse into his old difficulties with the c's and g's as in "crisis" and "give", the same two groups still seem to worry him: the "a" vowel, especially when it was followed by a consonant, as in "a-go" or "a-lone"

254

and a repeated sound or letter, as in the combination "yes please" or "Which we".'

That November brought another State Opening of Parliament—and another speech. Going through the text with the King, Logue played his habitual role of identifying and eliminating potential tongue twisters and other awkward phrases that might trip him up. 'In an unbreakable alliance' looked like it was going to cause problems, as did 'fortified by constant collaboration of the governments concerned'— so both were replaced. Another phrase, 'on windy beaches', was replaced by 'storm swept beaches'.

On the evening of Sunday 3 December the King was due to make a speech on the radio to mark the disbanding of the Home Guard, the two-million-strong defence force formed of men either too young, too old or too unfit to join the army. The force had been created in July 1940 to help defend Britain against a Nazi invasion, which appeared imminent. Now, in a reflection of the conviction that the tide of war had finally turned in the Allies' favour, it was being disbanded. Logue worked with the King on the text of the speech and went to Windsor to hear him speak. He was impressed to note he made only one mistake: he stumbled over the 'w' in weapons.

Afterwards, Logue shook hands with the King and, after congratulating him, asked why that particular letter had proved such a problem.

'I did it on purpose,' the King replied with a grin.

'On purpose?' asked Logue, incredulous.

'Yes. If I don't make a mistake, people might not know it was me.'

That Christmas, there was another message to the nation and on 23 December Logue went to Windsor to go over the wording. Its tone was optimistic—expressing the hope that before the following Christmas the nightmare of tyranny and conflict would be over. 'If we look back to those early days of the war, we can surely say that the darkness daily grows less and less,' the text read. 'The lamps which the Germans put out all over Europe, first in 1914 and then in 1939, are slowly being rekindled. Already we can see some of them beginning to shine through the fog of war that still surrounds so many lands. Anxiety is giving way to confidence and let us hope that before next Christmas Day, the story of liberation and triumph will be complete.'

An annotated copy of the text, found among Logue's papers, shows the changes he made to eliminate words or phrases that could still catch out the King: 'calamities', with that difficult initial 'k' sound, for example, was replaced by 'disasters', while 'goal', with its tricky 'g' at the beginning, was substituted by the much easier 'end'. All in all, though, Logue was impressed by the text. 'They all have to be cut out of the same pattern, but I think we altered this particular one less than any other,' he wrote.

As they sat in the study, with the fire burning, the King suddenly said: 'Logue, I think the time has come when I can do a broadcast by myself, and you can have a Christmas dinner with your family.'

Logue had been expecting this moment for some time, especially since the Home Guard speech. They discussed the matter thoroughly with the Queen, who agreed they should give it a try. So, instead of Logue, it was decided that, for the first time, she and the two princesses would sit beside the King at the microphone as he delivered his message.

'You know, Ma'am, I feel like a father who is sending his boy to his first public school,' Logue told the Queen as he went to go.

'I know just how you feel,' she replied, putting her hand on his arm and patting it.

Logue, spending his first Christmas at home for several years, celebrated with a house party; John Gordon of the *Sunday Express* and his wife were among the guests. Logue was so busy with all the preparations that he scarcely thought about the speech, but at five minutes to three he slipped off into his bedroom. After saying a silent prayer, he turned on the radio softly, just in time.

When the King's voice came through, Logue was astonished at how firm and resonant it was. It was three years since he had last heard him speak over the radio and he sounded much better than Logue remembered. He was speaking confidently and with good inflection and emphasis, and the breaks between words had all but disappeared. During the eight-minute message, he stopped only on one word, 'God', but it was only for a second and then he continued even more firmly than before.

Logue's guests had been listening in the drawing room and when he went back to join them, he was overwhelmed with congratulations.

He then tried a little joke: 'Would you like to hear the King speak?'

'Well, we've just heard him,' replied Gordon.

'If you go to the two extensions of the phone, you will hear him talk from Windsor.'

During their last run-through, it had been agreed that Logue would call the King after the speech; so he took the main phone and telephoned Windsor, while his guests listened in on the two extensions. A few seconds later, the King's voice came through.

Logue congratulated him on a wonderful talk, adding: 'My job is over, Sir.'

'Not at all,' the King replied. 'It is the preliminary work that counts, and that is where you are indispensable.'

The Christmas message was well received, and Logue received a number of letters of congratulations—including one from Hugh Crichton-Miller, a leading psychiatrist who had been based for some time at 146 Harley Street. 'That broadcast was streets ahead of any previous performance,' Crichton-Miller wrote to Logue on Boxing Day. 'One heard the self-expression of a new freedom which was wholly admirable.'

A delighted Logue passed it on to the King, who was flattered by the compliment—and had kind words for his teacher. 'I do hope you did not mind not being there as I felt that I just had to get one broadcast over alone,' he wrote back to Logue on 8 January. 'The preparation of speeches and broadcasts is the important part and that is where all your help is invaluable. I wonder if you realise how grateful I am to you for having made it possible for me to carry out this vital part of my job. I cannot thank you enough.'

Four days later, Logue responded, 'When we began years ago, the goal I set myself for you was to be able to make a speech without stumbling and talk over the air without fear of the microphone,'

258

he wrote. 'As you say, these things are now an accomplished fact, and I would not be human if I were not overjoyed that you can now do these things without supervision.

'When a fresh patient comes to me the usual query is: "Will I be able to speak like the King?" and my reply is: "Yes, if you will work like he does." I will cure anyone of intelligence if they will only work like you did—for you are now reaping the benefit of this tremendously hard work you did at the beginning.'

*   *   *

By January 1945 the Germans had been repulsed in the Ardennes without achieving any of their strategic objectives. The Soviets attacked in Poland, moving on to Silesia and Pomerania and advancing towards Vienna. The Western Allies, meanwhile, crossed the Rhine, north and south of the Ruhr, in March, and the following month pushed forward into Italy and swept across Western Germany. The two forces linked up on the River Elbe on May 25. Five days later, the capture of the Reichstag signalled the military defeat of the Third Reich. With Soviet troops only a few hundred yards away, Hitler shot himself in his bunker.

CHAPTER FIFTEEN

Victory

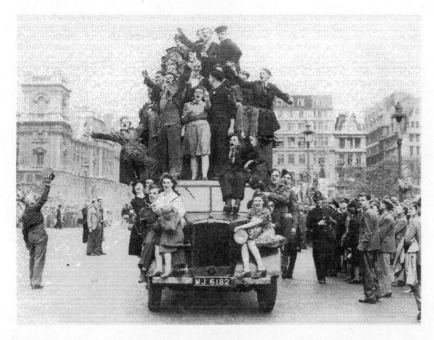

News of Germany's surrender in 1945 was met
with unbridled enthusiasm and relief

It was one of the greatest—and certainly the most joyous—street parties London had ever seen. On Tuesday 8 May 1945, tens of thousands of singing, dancing people gathered in the Mall in front of Buckingham Palace. The moment they had dreamed of for more than five and a half years had finally arrived.

The German surrender had been on the cards for several days: a team of bell ringers was on standby to ring in victory at St Paul's Cathedral, people stocked up on Union Jack flags and houses were garlanded with bunting. Then at three o'clock, Winston Churchill finally spoke to the nation: at 2.41 a.m. the previous day, he announced, the ceasefire had been signed by Colonel General Alfred Jodl, Chief of the Operations Staff of the Armed Forces High Command, at the American advance headquarters in Reims. In his speech, Churchill paid fulsome tribute to the men and women who had 'fought valiantly' on land, sea and in the air—and to those who had laid down their lives for victory. His broadcast was delivered from the War Cabinet Office, the same room in which his predecessor Neville Chamberlain had announced the country was at war six years earlier.

'We may allow ourselves a brief period of rejoicing,' Churchill concluded. 'But let us not forget for a moment the toil and efforts that lie ahead. Japan, with all her treachery and greed, remains unsubdued.'

Shortly afterwards, the King, as much a symbol of national resistance as Churchill, stepped out onto the balcony of Buckingham Palace to acknowledge the cheers of the ecstatic crowd below. For the first time in public, he was accompanied not just by the Queen but by the two princesses. At 5.30 p.m. the doors opened again, and the royal family stepped out once more—this time together with Churchill. They were to make a total of eight such appearances that day. Later that evening, the King was due to follow his prime minister in addressing the nation.

At 11.30 a.m. on the previous Saturday, Logue had received a telephone call from Lascelles asking him to go to Windsor that afternoon: 'Peace Day V', as it was known, was in the offing. Lascelles was still not certain of the exact day; it all depended on what happened in Norway. The German forces occupying the country had contemplated turning it into a last bastion of the Third Reich, but had finally come to realize the futility of further resistance. The only question was when they would capitulate. A car came to Sydenham Hill to pick up Logue, and he was at Windsor Castle by 4 p.m.

He arrived to find the King looking completely exhausted. They went through the speech, which Logue really liked—although they altered a few passages. They had a further run-through, this time at Buckingham Palace, on Monday at 3 p.m., and it was agreed that Logue should return at 8.30 that evening. He went home for a rest, but at six o'clock the telephone range; it was Lascelles. 'Not tonight,' he said. 'Norway has not come into line.' But he assured Logue this was certain the following night and told him to stand by.

The next morning Logue received another

message from the Palace. 'The King would like to see you at dinner tonight, and bring Mrs Logue'—to which someone had added the cryptic message: 'Tell her to wear something bright'. So at 6.30 p.m., Lionel and Myrtle set off towards Buckingham Palace. The streets were virtually deserted and it took them only a few minutes to drive into the centre of London. They encountered the first traffic barrier near Victoria Station, but Mieville had organized a permit, and they continued on their way towards the Palace. As their car crossed the courtyard towards the Privy Purse entrance, a tremendous cheer broke out—the King and Queen had just come out again onto the balcony. Lionel and Myrtle joined other members of the royal household in wildly cheering and waving handkerchiefs.

Lionel made for the new broadcasting room on the ground floor, facing the lawn, and went through the speech with the King. They made a couple of alterations, more for the running of the speech than anything else, and then the King, rather plaintively, declared, 'If I don't get dinner before nine I won't get any after, as everyone will be away, watching the sights.' This, coming from a man in such an exalted position, sent Logue into paroxysms of laughter—so much so that the King himself joined in; but after thinking it over, he said, 'It's funny, but it is quite true.'

After they had eaten, they went back to the broadcasting room at 8.35. Wood of the BBC was there; he and Logue compared watches and they had another run-through. There were two minutes to go. Another small further alteration and then, as usual, the Queen, who was dressed in white, came in to wish her husband luck. As the floodlights were switched on, a mighty roar erupted from the crowd. Logue found the atmosphere fantastic: 'And in an instant the sombre scene has become fairyland—with the Royal Ensign, lit from beneath, floating in the air,' he wrote in his diary. 'Another roar—the King and Queen come on to the balcony.' He was especially struck by the way the lights played on the Queen's tiara; as she turned, smiling, to wave to the crowd, the floodlights created what looked like a band of flame around her head. The King declared:

Today we give thanks to Almighty God for a great deliverance. Speaking from our Empire's oldest capital city, war-battered but never for one moment daunted or dismayed, speaking from London, I ask you to join with me in that act of thanksgiving.

Germany, the enemy who drove all Europe into war, has been finally overcome. In the Far East we have yet to deal with the Japanese, a determined and cruel foe. To this we shall turn with the utmost resolve and with all our resources. But at this hour when the dreadful shadow of war has passed far from our hearths and homes in these islands, we may at last make one pause for thanksgiving and then turn our thoughts to the task all over the world which peace in Europe brings with it.

Continuing, the King saluted those who had contributed to victory—both alive and dead—and reflected on how the 'enslaved and isolated peoples of Europe' had looked to Britain during the darkest days of the conflict. He also looked to the future, urging that Britons should 'resolve as a people to do nothing unworthy of those who died for us and to make the world such a world as they would have desired, for their children and for ours. This is the task to which now honour binds us,' he concluded. 'In the hour of danger we humbly committed our cause into the Hand of God, and He has been our Strength and Shield. Let us thank him for his mercies, and in this hour of Victory commit ourselves and our new guidance of that same strong Hand.'

The King was exhausted, and it showed; he stumbled more than usual over his words, but it didn't seem to matter. 'We all roared ourselves hoarse,' recalled Noël Coward, who was among the crowd. 'I suppose this is the greatest day in our history.'

As the celebrations continued, the two princesses asked their parents for permission to be allowed out into the throng. The King agreed: 'Poor darlings, they have never had any fun yet,' he wrote in his diary. And so, at 10.30 p.m., accompanied by a discreet escort of Guards officers, Elizabeth and Margaret slipped out of the Palace incognito. No one seems to have recognized the two young women as they joined the conga line into one door of the Ritz and out of the other.

At 11.30 the Queen sent for Lionel and Myrtle, and they said their goodbyes. Then Peter Townsend, the King's equerry and future lover of Princess Margaret, led them out through the gardens to the Royal Mews where a car was waiting for them. The crowds had thinned considerably by then, but there were still plenty of people out on the streets celebrating victory.

As the Logues drove home, they gave a ride as far as the Kennington Oval, in south London, to a soldier and then, after he got out, to a couple with a little girl, who wanted to go to Dog Kennel Hill which was near their home. As they drove, they talked about the evening's events and about the King and Queen. The couple thanked the Logues warmly as they got out; Lionel heard the baby's sleepy little voice saying goodnight.

*   *   *

Although Logue had recently celebrated his sixty-fifth birthday, he had no plans for retirement and continued to see other patients. On 3 June 1945, Mieville wrote to thank him for 'what you did for young Astor'—a reference to Michael Astor, the twenty-nine-year-old son of Viscount Astor, the wealthy owner of the *Observer* newspaper, who wanted to follow his father into politics. 'Your efforts were successful in that he was adopted for his constituency,' Mieville added. 'He ought to get in as it is a v. safe seat, but I fear he will not contribute much when he does arrive in the House of Commons.' Astor was duly elected as the Member of Parliament for Surrey East in the following month's general election, but served only until 1951 and made little impact on British public life.

For Logue, joy at the return of peace was soon to be tinged with personal tragedy.

That June he was in St Andrew's Hospital in Dollis Hill in north-west London having an operation on his prostate when Myrtle suffered a

268

heart attack and was taken to the same hospital. She died a few days later on 22 June.

Lionel was heartbroken. During their more than forty years together, Myrtle had been a dominant figure in his life; they had been deeply in love. During an appearance in 1942 on a BBC programme called *On My Selection*—similar to today's *Desert Island Discs*—he had described his wife as 'the lass who has stood by my side . . . and helped me so valiantly over the rough places'. She was cremated at Honor Oak Crematorium in south-east London, near their home.

The King sent a telegram of condolence as soon as he heard the news: 'The Queen and I are grieved to hear of Mrs Logue's death and send you and your family our deepest sympathy in your loss—George.' He followed up with two letters: one on 27 June and a second on the following day. 'I was so shocked when I was told because your wife was in such good form on Victory night,' he wrote. 'Please do not hesitate to let me know if I can be of any help to you.'

Logue had to face his grief without two of his three sons: Valentine was due to leave a few weeks later for India with a neuro-surgical unit, while Tony seemed likely to be sent back to Italy. He hoped at least Laurie would remain in Britain, though. 'He has had a bad time in Africa and has not yet recovered,' he wrote to the King on 14 July. 'I don't know quite what I would have done without him.'

Logue's own health continued to be poor, but he nevertheless went back to work, 'the great panacea for all sorrow'. 'I am entirely at your Majesty's command,' he added. 'I expect there will be a

Parliament to be opened shortly.'

The State Opening, which took place on 15 August, saw a return to the pomp of pre-war years, with thousands of people lining the streets of London as the King and Queen travelled to parliament in the royal coach. There was an extra cause for celebration: earlier that day, following America's dropping of atomic bombs on Hiroshima and Nagasaki, Emperor Hirohito of Japan announced his country's surrender. The Second World War was finally over.

In content, the speech written for the King was one of the most dramatic for decades. That July's election had for the first time returned a Labour government with an absolute majority—and a mandate for a programme of sweeping social, economic and political change that would transform the face of Britain. Among the major reforms to which the new administration was committed was the nationalization of the mines, the railways, the Bank of England and the gas and electricity companies, as well as reform of the welfare and education systems and the creation of the National Health Service. 'It will be the aim of my ministers to see that national resources in labour and material are employed with the fullest efficiency in the interests of all,' the King declared.

A natural conservative, the King was concerned at the potential impact of some of his new government's more radical measures. He was also saddened by the defeat of Churchill, with whom he had formed a close bond during the war. Yet whatever his misgivings, he was a constitutional monarch and had no alternative but to accept his new government. On a personal level, he developed good relations with Clement Attlee, the prime minister—like the King a man of few words—as well as with several of the new Labour ministers. He had something of a natural affinity with Aneurin Bevan, the minister of health, even though he was a member of the Labour left. Bevan, too, had long suffered with a stammer and told the King during his first audience of his admiration for the way he had overcome his speech defect.

*   *   *

Although the war had ended, life remained tough for ordinary Britons; the economy had been dealt a serious blow from which it would take many years to recover. Rationing, far from being ended, actually became stricter: bread, which had been freely on sale during the war, was rationed from 1946 until 1948; potato rationing was introduced for the first time in 1947. It was not until 1954 that rationing was finally abolished, with meat and bacon the last items to go.

Logue continued with his practice. 'Life goes on, and I am working very hard, harder than I should have [to at] my age 66, but work is the only thing that lets me forget,' he wrote in a letter to Myrtle's brother, Rupert, in May 1946. In the letter he expressed the hope that he could go back to Australia for six months, in what would have been his first trip home since he and Myrtle emigrated to Britain in 1924. He was suffering from abnormally high blood pressure, however, and was warned by the doctors not to fly. This meant having to wait until normal shipping services resumed. He never made the trip.

Of Logue's various cases, particularly poignant was that of Jack Fennell, a thirty-one-year-old stammerer from Merthyr Tydfil in Wales, who in September 1947 had written to the King pleading for his assistance. Unemployed, penniless and with a child to feed, Fennell was despondent and suffered from an inferiority complex brought on by years of discrimination over his stammer. Lascelles forwarded Fennell's letter to Logue on 24 September, asking him to take a look at him and give an opinion on his condition. Logue reckoned he might need as much as a year of treatment, which Fennell couldn't afford. After trying in vain to get help from the various welfare bodies, Fennell eventually found a sponsor in Viscount Kemsley, the newspaper baron who owned the *Daily Sketch* and *The Sunday Times*. With lodging in an army hostel in Westminster and the offer of a job at the Kemsley newspaper press in London, Fennell began his treatment in January 1948.

By April the following year, Logue was able to write back to Kemsley boasting of the progress his patient had made: Fennell had grown in confidence and passed 'with flying colours' an interview to work at the Atomic Energy Research Establishment at Harwell. Logue continued to see him for another year, although their appointments were reduced to just one a month. By August 1949, things were going so well at work that Fennell had moved his family into a house in Wantage; in January the following year he enrolled at the Oxford College of Technology and by May was offered a permanent job at Harwell.

*   *   *

With Myrtle gone and his sons now grown, Logue sold the house on Sydenham Hill in April 1947. It was not just that it was far too big for him now; as he wrote to the King that December in his annual birthday greetings, 'it held too many memories' of his decades of married life. He moved to 29 Princes Court, a 'comfortable little flat' in the Brompton Road in Knightsbridge, just opposite Harrods.

There were more problems at home. Tony, Lionel's youngest, had in the meantime left the army and returned to university, only this time it was Cambridge. He continued to study medicine for nine months, but his heart was not in it and he switched to law. He was in delicate health, however. He went into hospital for a relatively straightforward operation on his appendix, but then had to have four major operations within six days. In his customary birthday letter to the King, Logue blamed the dramatic turn of events on a delayed reaction to an incident when his son was serving in North Africa and was unconscious for four days after getting too close to an explosion. Tony had been involved 'in a desperate fight for his life', he wrote. The King wrote back two days later expressing sympathy. 'You have certainly had your share of shocks and sorrows,' he said. As usual, he updated Logue on his public speaking, noting how pleased he was with a speech he had made at his father's memorial. He expressed concern, however, that his Christmas message would not be easy, 'because everything is so

273

gloomy'.

Logue did, however, see one ambition realized: on 19 January 1948, he wrote to the King asking him to become patron of the College of Speech Therapists, which now counted 350 members, was 'quite solvent' and was now recognized by the British Medical Association. 'I am sixty-eight years of age and it will be a wonderful thought in my old age to know that you were the head of this rapidly growing and essential organisation,' he wrote. The King agreed.

Logue was still finding it difficult to come to terms with Myrtle's death. They had been married for almost forty years, during which she had been a dominant influence on him, and her death left a massive hole in his life. Although otherwise a rational man, he became attracted to spiritualism in the hope of making contact with her on the 'other side'. As a result he got in touch with Lilian Bailey, a 'deep trance medium'. Over the years, Bailey had been consulted by a number of prominent figures in Britain and abroad—among them the Hollywood actresses Mary Pickford, Merle Oberon and Mae West, and Mackenzie King, the Canadian prime minister.

Quite how Logue got in touch with Bailey and how many séances he attended is unclear; his sons, however, were appalled when he used to tell them he was going off to 'get in touch' with his late wife. 'It was something we thought was really crazy and wished to goodness he wasn't doing it,' recalled Valentine Logue's wife Anne.[90]

*　　*　　*

Amid the gloom of the immediate post-war years, there was one glimmer of light: on 10 July 1947, it was announced that Princess Elizabeth would marry Philip, the son of Prince Andrew of Greece and Denmark and the British-born Princess Alice of Battenberg. The couple had met in June 1939 when Philip was eighteen and the future Queen just thirteen. The King had travelled with his family on the Royal Yacht to visit the Royal Naval College at Dartmouth, and during the visit someone had to look after Elizabeth and Margaret, then aged nine.

Lord Mountbatten, the King's ambitious aide-de-camp, made sure that of all the young men present, it was his nephew Philip, a tall, strikingly good-looking man who had just graduated as the top cadet in his course, who was given the task. Elizabeth (who was Philip's third cousin through Queen Victoria, and second cousin, once removed, through Christian IX of Denmark) was smitten. 'Lilibet never took her eyes off him,' observed Marion Crawford, her governess, in her memoirs. The couple soon began to exchange letters.

What appeared to have started as a crush on Princess Elizabeth's part soon turned to a full-blown romance—which was encouraged at every stage by Mountbatten, who was keen to see his family linked with the House of Windsor. Elizabeth and Philip wrote to each other and even managed occasional meetings when Philip was on leave, but so long as the war continued, there was little chance of their relationship going any further. That was changed by the outbreak of peace.

The King had mixed feelings about the match,

not least because he considered his daughter too young and was concerned she had fallen for the first young man she had ever met. Philip was also seen by many at court—the King included—as far from the ideal consort for a future monarch, not least because of his German blood; the Queen was said to refer to him privately as 'the Hun'. Hoping their daughter might find someone else, she and the King organized a series of balls packed with eligible men, to which Philip, to his great annoyance, was not invited. Yet Elizabeth remained devoted to her prince.

Eventually, in 1946, Philip asked the King for his daughter's hand in marriage. George agreed—but still had one last trick up his sleeve: he insisted any formal announcement was postponed until after Elizabeth's twenty-first birthday the following April. By the month before, at Mountbatten's suggestion, Philip had renounced his Greek and Danish titles, as well as his allegiance to the Greek crown, converted from Greek Orthodoxy to the Church of England and become a naturalized British subject. He also adopted the surname Mountbatten (an Anglicized version of Battenberg) from his mother's family.

The couple married on 20 November 1947 in Westminster Abbey in a ceremony attended by representatives of various royal families—but not Philip's three surviving sisters, who had married German aristocrats with Nazi connections. On the morning of the wedding, Philip was made Duke of Edinburgh, Earl of Merioneth and Baron Greenwich of Greenwich in the County of London; the previous day the King had bestowed on him the style of His Royal Highness.

The King's public speaking may have been getting better and better, but his health was getting worse. He was still only forty-nine when the war ended, but he was in poor physical shape: the strain he suffered during the war is often given as a prime reason, yet it is difficult to see how this strain was any greater than that suffered by the millions of men who served on the front line or indeed by the civilian population left behind. Another factor was his chain-smoking: in July 1941 *Time* magazine reported that, in order to share the hardship of his people, he was cutting down from twenty or twenty-five cigarettes a day to a mere fifteen. After the war, he started smoking more again.

Despite his poor health, the King set off in February 1947 on a ten-week tour of South Africa. He had already been to Australia, New Zealand and Canada, but had never visited South Africa and was keen to see it. The itinerary was a gruelling one and the King tired easily; a warm reception from the Afrikaners, especially from those old enough to remember the Boer War, was by no means guaranteed. There was also an added psychological strain: Britain was in the grip of one of the bitterest winters for decades, and the King suffered pangs of guilt at not sharing his subjects' suffering. At one point he even suggested cutting short his trip, although Attlee strongly advised against it, warning that this would only add to the sense of crisis.

Within two months of his return, the King was beginning to suffer cramp in his legs, complaining in a letter to Logue of 'feeling tired and strained'.[91] By October 1948 these cramps had become painful and permanent: his left foot was numb all day and the pain kept him awake all night; later, the problem seemed to shift to the right. The King was examined the following month by Professor James Learmonth, one of Britain's greatest authorities on vascular complaints, who found him to be suffering from early arteriosclerosis; at one stage it was feared that the King's right leg might have to be amputated because of the possibility of gangrene. A few weeks later Logue wrote to express his concerns: 'As one who had the honour to be closely connected with you during those dreadful war years and had a glimpse of the enormous amount of work you did, and saw the strain that was constantly made on your vitality, it is very evident that you have driven yourself too hard and at last have had to call a halt,' he wrote on 24 November. 'I know that rest, medical skill and your own wonderful spirit will restore you to health.'

The King appeared to have recovered by December, but the doctors ordered continued rest, and a trip to Australia and New Zealand planned for early the next year had to be abandoned. The King nevertheless seemed upbeat in a letter to Logue on 10 December. 'I am getting better with treatment and rest in bed, and the doctors do have a smile on their face, which I feel is all to the good,' he wrote. 'I hope you are well & are still helping those who cannot speak.'

Lionel, who was fifteen years the King's senior, was also having a bad year—and was confined for some of the time to his new flat, which was on the eighth floor. As he wrote in his annual birthday letter to the King that December, he was in such poor health that friends wrote home to Australia saying they didn't think he would survive. He was heartened, though, by the apparent good news about the King's condition. 'I have followed the wonderful struggle you have made and rejoice the Almighty has brought you back to health,' he wrote.

Christmas was looming—and with it the annual message. 'I have got a new type of broadcast this year from a more personal angle which I hope will go well,' the King wrote to Logue on the twentieth. In a sign of the progress he had made over the years, he no longer looked to Logue to help him prepare for his broadcast, as he had in the old days, although he urged him to telephone afterwards to give his opinion on his performance.

The King delivered the message from Sandringham, returning to London only at the end of February, when he resumed a limited programme of audiences and held an investiture. March 1949 brought bad news, however. After a full examination, it was decided the King's recovery had not been as complete as everyone had thought; Learmonth advised a right lumbar sympathectomy, a surgical procedure intended to free the flow of blood to his leg. The operation, which was carried out at the King's insistence in an impromptu operating theatre in Buckingham Palace rather than a hospital, went well. The King was under no illusions, however, that he would be completely restored to health; his doctors ordered him to rest, reduce his official engagements and cut down drastically on the smoking that had aggravated his condition; a second attack of thrombosis could be lethal.

The King's health appeared to continue to improve through 1949, but the doctors nevertheless ordered as much rest as possible. That Christmas brought another message to the nation, the Commonwealth and the Empire. 'Once more I am in the throes of preparing my broadcast,' the King wrote to Logue, thanking him for his annual birthday greetings. 'How difficult it is to find anything new to say in these days. Words of encouragement to do better in the New Year is the only thing to go on. I am longing to get it over. It still ruins my Christmas.'

CHAPTER SIXTEEN

The Last Words

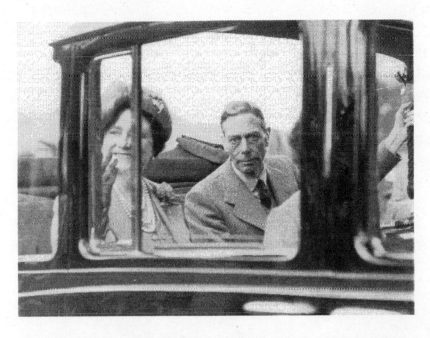

George VI looking tired and ill shortly before
his death

To the millions of people in Britain and across the Commonwealth and Empire who gathered around their radios on Christmas Day 1951, the voice was both familiar and yet worryingly different. George VI was delivering his traditional Christmas message, but he sounded uncomfortably husky and hoarse, as if he were suffering from a particularly heavy cold. At times, his voice dropped to almost a whisper. He also seemed to be speaking slightly faster than usual. Yet few of those listening could have failed to be moved by what their monarch had to say.

After beginning by describing Christmas as a time when everyone should count their blessings, the King struck a deeply personal note.

I myself have every cause for deep thankfulness, for not only—by the grace of God and through the faithful skill of my doctors, surgeons and nurses—have I come through my illness, but I have learned once again that it is in bad times that we value most highly the support and sympathy of our friends. From my peoples in these islands and in the British Commonwealth and Empire as well as from many other countries this support and sympathy has reached me and I thank you now from my heart. I trust that you yourselves realise how greatly your prayers and good wishes have helped and are helping me in my recovery.

The King's five doctors telephoned their

congratulations, but the newspapers both in Britain and beyond were shocked by what they heard. Although commentators and leader writers were relieved to hear the King speak for the first time since a major operation three months earlier, the wavering tone of his voice brought home to them quite how poorly he was. 'Millions of people all over the world, listening to the King's Christmas Day broadcast, noticed with concern the huskiness in his voice,' the *Daily Mirror* reported two days later. 'The question at many Christmas firesides was: Is the King just suffering from a chill, or is the huskiness a sequel to the lung operation he had three months ago?'

For the first time since he had delivered his first Christmas message in 1937, the King's words were not being spoken live—as Sir John Reith had always insisted they should be during his long tenure as director-general of the BBC—but had been pre-recorded. The explanation for this innovation lay in the further worsening of the King's health.

After the various medical crises he suffered in the late 1940s, the King had been ordered by his doctors to rest and relax as much as possible and to cut down his public appearances. A further strain on his health came from the worsening economic and political situation: Attlee's Labour party, elected by a landslide in 1945, had seen its majority eroded to a handful in 1950 and was struggling to continue in office. A general election in October 1951 brought a change of government with the return of the seventy-six-year-old Winston Churchill.

The King had been well enough to open the

Festival of Britain on 3 May, riding with the Queen in an open carriage through the streets of London, escorted by the Household Cavalry. 'This is no time for despondency,' he announced from the steps of St Paul's Cathedral. 'I see this festival as a symbol of Britain's abiding courage and vitality.' But many who saw their monarch close up during the service remarked on how ill he looked—and that evening he took to his bed with influenza.

The King was slow to recover and also suffered from a persistent cough; he was initially diagnosed with a catarrhal inflammation of the left lung and treated with penicillin. The symptoms persisted, but it was not until 15 September that he was found to have a malignant growth. Three days later, Clement Price Thomas, a surgeon who specialized in such problems, told the King the lung should be removed as soon as possible—although, as was the practice of the day, he did not reveal to his patient that he was suffering from cancer.

The operation, carried out on 23 September, went well. It had been feared that the King might lose certain nerves in the larynx, which could mean he would be unable to speak in more than a whisper. The fear proved unfounded. By October he was writing to his mother expressing relief that he had not suffered complications.

He was nevertheless still a sick man. During the State Opening of Parliament that November, his speech from the throne—exceptionally—was read for him by Lord Simonds, the Lord Chancellor. There were suggestions that he should step aside for the Christmas broadcast as well. According to one later newspaper report,[92] it was proposed that his place at the microphone be taken by his wife or by Princess Elizabeth. This would certainly have spared the King considerable discomfort, but he refused. 'My daughter may have her opportunity next Christmas,' he told them. 'I want to speak to my people myself.' The King's determination to deliver his message in person—much as he had always dreaded doing so—showed the extent to which, during the course of his reign, those few minutes on the afternoon of 25 December had been turned into one of the most important events in the national calendar.

The doctors warned, however, that a live broadcast could prove too much of a strain, so a compromise was found: the King recorded the message in sections, sentence by sentence, repeating some over and over again, until he was satisfied. The finished result was barely six minutes long, but recording it took the best part of two days. It was far from perfect: what seemed to listeners an uncharacteristically fast delivery appears to have been one of the side effects of the editing process. As far as the King was concerned, though, it was far better than any of the alternatives. 'The nation will hear my message, although it might have been better,' he told the sound engineer and a senior official from the BBC, who were the only two people allowed to listen back with him to the final version before it was broadcast. 'Thank you for your patience.'

The letter that the King sent Logue in response to his customary birthday greetings on 14 December reflected quite how low he had been feeling in the run-up to the recording. It was to be the last letter that he wrote to his speech therapist

286

and friend, and his remarks seemed all the more poignant because Logue himself was also in poor health.

I am so sorry to hear that you have not been well again,' the King wrote. 'As for myself, I have spent a wretched year culminating in that very severe operation, from which I seem to be making a remarkable recovery. The latter fact is in many ways entirely down to you. Before this operation, Price Thomas the surgeon asked to see me breathe. When he saw the diaphragm move up and down naturally he asked me whether I had always breathed in that way. I said no, I had been taught to breathe like that in 1926 & had gone on doing so. Another feather in your cap you see!!

Logue wanted to reply, but he was taken into hospital before he could respond.

*   *   *

The King stayed on at Sandringham into the New Year with the Queen. The note of hope and confidence in his Christmas speech appeared to be justified. He was well enough to begin shooting again, and when he was examined by his doctors on 29 January, they pronounced themselves satisfied with his recovery. The next day the royal family went to the theatre at Drury Lane to see *South Pacific*. The outing had something of an air of celebration about it, partly because of the improvement in the King's health and partly because, the following day, Princess Elizabeth and the Duke of Edinburgh were due to set off for East Africa, Australia and New Zealand.

On 5 February, a cold, but dry and sunny day, the King enjoyed a day of shooting. He was, according to his official biographer, 'as carefree and happy as those about him had ever known him'.[93] After a relaxed dinner, he retired to his room and, about midnight, went to bed. At 7.30 the following morning, a servant found him dead in his bed. The cause of death was not cancer, but rather a coronary thrombosis—a fatal blood clot to the heart—that he suffered soon after falling asleep.

By this time, Elizabeth and Philip had reached the Kenyan stage of their trip: they had just returned to Sagana Lodge, one hundred miles north of Nairobi, after a night spent at Treetops Hotel, when word arrived of the King's death; it fell to Philip to break the news to his wife. She was proclaimed Queen and the royal party quickly returned to Britain.

On 26 February Logue wrote to the King's widow, who, at the age of fifty-one had begun what was to be more than half a century as Queen Mother. He referred to the 'wonderful letter' that her late husband had sent in December and expressed his regrets that his own illness had prevented him from replying to it—until it was too late. 'Since 1926 he honoured me, by allowing me to help him with his speech, & no man ever worked as hard as he did, & achieved such a grand result,' Logue wrote. 'During all those years you were a tower of strength to him & he has often told me how much he has owed to you, and the excellent result could never have been achieved if it had not been for your help. I have never forgotten your gracious help to me after my own beloved girl passed on.'

In her reply two days later, the Queen Mother was equally fulsome in her praise of Logue. 'I think that I know perhaps better than anyone just how much you helped the King, not only with his speech, but through that his whole life & outlook on life,' she wrote. 'I shall always be deeply grateful to you for all you did for him. He was such a splendid person and I don't believe that he ever thought of himself at all. I did so hope that he might have been allowed a few years of comparative peace after the many anguished years he has had to battle through so bravely. But it was not to be. I do hope that you will soon be better.'

That May, her daughter, now Queen Elizabeth II, mindful of how close Logue had been to her father, sent him a small gold snuff box that had belonged to the King, together with the following message:

I am sending you this little box which always stood on the King's table, & which he was rather fond of, as I am sure you would like a little personal souvenir of someone who was so grateful to you for all you did for him. The box was on his writing table, & I know that he would wish you to have it.

I do hope that you are feeling better. I miss the King more & more.

Yours v sincerely

Elizabeth R.

That December, the Queen gave her first Christmas message from Sandringham. 'Each Christmas, at this time, my beloved father broadcast a message to his people in all parts of the world,' she began. 'As he used to do, I am speaking to you from my own home, where I am spending Christmas with my family.' Speaking in clear, firm tones—and without a trace of the impediment that had so clouded her father's life— she paid tribute to those still serving in the armed forces abroad and thanked her subjects for the 'loyalty and affection' they had shown her since her accession to the throne ten months earlier. 'My father and my grandfather before him, worked hard all their lives to unite our peoples ever more closely, and to maintain its ideals which were so near to their hearts,' she said. 'I shall strive to carry on their work.'

Logue did not record what he thought of the speech—or indeed whether he listened to it, at all. Either way, his services were no longer required and his health was failing. He spent the festivities in his flat surrounded by his three sons and their families: Valentine and his wife Anne, with their two-year-old daughter, Victoria; Laurie and Jo, with their children, Alexandra, 14, and Robert, 10, and Antony, with his future wife Elizabeth, whom he would marry less than a year later.

Shortly after New Year, Logue was taken ill for the last time. He remained bedridden for more than three months, and a live-in nurse was employed to look after him, but he eventually fell into a coma. He died on 12 April 1953 of kidney failure, less than two months after his seventy-third birthday. Among his effects were two invitations to the Queen's coronation, to be held that June—the second presumably sent because he had been too sick to respond to the first.

The obituaries that appeared in Britain, Australia and America were brief. 'Mr Lionel Logue, C.V.O., who died yesterday at the age of 73, was one of the leading specialists in the treatment of speech defects and was mainly responsible for helping King George VI to overcome the impediment in his speech,' wrote *The Times*, which sandwiched him between the former president of Poland and the head of an American engineering company. 'He was on close personal terms with the King for a long time.' As for his techniques, the obituary writer merely noted: 'An important part of Logue's method was his instruction in how to breathe properly and so produce speed without strain.'

A few days later, readers added their comments: 'May I be allowed, through the courtesy of your columns, to pay a humble tribute to the great work of Mr Lionel Logue,' wrote a Mr J. C. Wimbusch. 'As a patient of his in 1926, I can testify to the fact that his patience was magnificent and his sympathy almost superhuman. It was at his house in Bolton Gardens that I was introduced to the late King, then Duke of York. There must be thousands of people who, like myself, are living to bless the name of Lionel Logue.'[94]

Logue's funeral was held on 17 April at Holy Trinity Church, Brompton. He was cremated. Both the Queen and the Queen Mother sent representatives, as did the Australian High

291

Commissioner. While Logue's work with the King had brought him prominence and honours—although strangely, given the closeness of their relationship, not a knighthood—it had not made him a wealthy man. In his will, details of which were published in *The Times* on 6 October, he left a fairly modest £8,605—the equivalent of about £180,000 today.

*   *   *

Even with the benefit of more than half a century's worth of hindsight, establishing quite how Logue succeeded with the King where those who preceded him had failed still remains something of a challenge. The various breathing exercises on which he put such emphasis certainly appear to have helped—the King, for one, appears to have been convinced of that. Important, too, was the effort that Logue put into going through the texts of the various speeches that had been written for him, removing words and phrases that he knew could potentially trip up his royal pupil. In a sense, though, this was not so much curing the problem, as avoiding it—yet there seems little doubt that by eliminating the largest of such stumbling blocks, Logue helped to build up the King's confidence, ensuring that the speech as a whole, with all the other lesser challenges it contained, proved less daunting.

Ultimately, though, the crucial factor appears to have been the way in which Logue, from the start, managed to persuade his patient that his was no deep seated psychological affliction, but rather an almost mechanical problem that could be

292

overcome through hard work and determination. An important part of this was the closeness of the relationship that developed between the two men, which was helped by Logue's no-nonsense approach. By insisting from the beginning that they should meet in his practice at Harley Street or at his own home, rather than on royal territory, Logue had made clear his intention that the King should be his patient; over the years this was to turn into a genuine friendship.

That being said, the two men's very different positions in what was still a very class-ridden society meant that there were limits to how close this relationship could be—especially after Bertie became King. The tone, not just of Logue's letters but also of entries in his diary, both of which have been quoted extensively in this book, reveal a deep respect not just for thc King as a person but also for the institution of monarchy. Indeed, to a modern reader, the tone Logue adopts when writing of thc King can seem fawning—especially more so in the case of the Queen Mother.

The last word belongs to one of the few people still alive at the time of writing who actually knew Logue well—his daughter-in-law Anne, who was married to his middle son Valentine, and who, in the summer of 2010, although already in her early nineties, remained enviably sharp and sprightly. Her opinions appeared to be given further weight by her career, which had culminated in her becoming Consultant in Child Psychiatry at the Middlesex Undergraduate Teaching Hospital.

Asked about the secret of her father-in-law's success, Anne, too, was unable to give a definitive answer, but thought it was largely due to the rapport that Logue had developed with the future King when his patient was still a young man, rather than to any particular treatment. 'Anyone can do tongue twisters and breathing exercises, but he was a first class psychotherapist,' she said. 'He was a super good daddy where George V had been a ghastly one.'

'[Lionel] would never talk about what he did. But when you look at what happened and what he was dealing with, that can be the only answer. The King had heaps of other people who had been no use to him. Why else did he stay with him for such a long time?'

The King's letter is in front of me as I write, & I cannot realize, that is so the last one, I shall ever receive. Since 1926 he honoured me, by allowing me to help him with his speech, & no man ever worked as hard as he did, & achieved such a grand result.

Notes

1 John W. Wheeler-Bennett, *King George VI, His Life and Reign*, London: Macmillan, 1958, p. 400.
2 *Ibid.*, p. 312.
3 *Time*, 16 May 1938.
4 Quoted in Joy Damousi, ' "The Australian has a lazy way of talking": Australian Character and Accent, 1920s–1940s', in Joy Damousi and Desley Deacon (eds), *Talking and Listening in the Age of Modernity: Essays on the History of Sound*, Canberra: ANU Press, 2007, pp. 83–96.
5 Lionel Logue papers, 25 March 1911.
6 *Sunday Times* (Perth), 20 August 1911.
7 *West Australian*, 27 May 1912.
8 *Sun* (Kalgoorlie), 27 September 1914.
9 The following dialogue is taken from an account by John Gordon in the *Sunday Express*.
10 Marcel E. Wingate, *Stuttering: A Short History of a Curious Disorder*, Westport, CT: Bergin & Garvey, 1997, p.11.
11 *Ibid.*, p. xx.
12 *Star*, 11 January 1926.
13 *Pittsburgh Press*, 1 December 1928.
14 Reported in the *Daily Express*, Friday 21 August 1925 and reproduced in full in *Radio Times* on 25 September. The BBC became the British Broadcasting Corporation only in 1926.
15 John Gore, *King George V*, London: John Murray.
16 Sarah Bradford, *The Reluctant King: The Life and Reign of George VI 1895–1952*, New York: St Martin's Press, 1990, p.18.
17 *Ibid.*, p. 18.

18 *Ibid.*, p. 22.
19 *Ibid.*, p. 40.
20 *Ibid.*, p. 33.
21 Wheeler-Bennett, *op. cit.*, p. 42.
22 Bradford, *op. cit.*, p. 48.
23 Lambert and Hamilton quoted in *ibid.*, p. 57.
24 *Ibid.*, p. 70.
25 Robert Rhodes James, *A Spirit Undaunted: The Political Role Of George VI*, London: Little, Brown, 1998, p. 92.
26 Davidson papers quoted in *ibid.*, p. 96.
27 *Pittsburgh Press*, 1 December 1928.
28 Wheeler-Bennett, *op. cit.*, p. 207.
29 *Ibid.*, p. 208.
30 *Ibid.*
31 Taylor Darbyshire, *The Duke of York: an intimate & authoritative life-story of the second son of their majesties, the King and Queen by one who has had special facilities, and published with the approval of his Royal Highness*, London: Hutchinson and Co., 1929, p. 90.
32 Michael Thornton, email correspondence with the author, July 2010.
33 Darbyshire, *op.cit.*, p. 22.
34 *Scotsman*, 2 December 1926.
35 Lionel Logue papers, 5 January 1927.
36 Wheeler-Bennett, *op. cit.*, p. 215.
37 *Ibid.*, p. 216.
38 Lionel Logue papers, 25 January 1927.
39 *Ibid.*, 14 February 1927.
40 Wheeler-Bennett, *op. cit.*, p. 218.
41 Reginald Pound, *Harley Street*, London: Michael Joseph, 1967, p. 157.
42 Wheeler-Bennett, *op. cit.*, p. 227.
43 *Ibid.*, p. 228.

44 *Ibid.*, p. 230.
45 Lionel Logue papers.
46 Wheeler-Bennett, *op. cit.*, p. 230.
47 Lionel Logue papers.
48 *Ibid.*
49 Pound, *op. cit.*, p. 157.
50 *Evening Standard* (London), 12 June 1928; *North-Eastern Daily Gazette*, 13 July 1928; *Evening News* (London), 24 October 1928; *Daily Sketch*, 28 November 1928; *Yorkshire Evening News*, 4 December 1928.
51 Lionel Logue papers, 15 December 1928.
52 Wheeler-Bennett, *op. cit.*, p. 251.
53 This and the following extracts from the Logue–Duke correspondence in the Lionel Logue papers.
54 Wheeler-Bennett, *op. cit.*, p. 258.
55 Lionel Logue papers, 12 February 1929.
56 *Ibid.*, 16 and 23 May 1934.
57 Wheeler-Bennett, *op. cit.*, p. 263.
58 James Lees-Milne, *The Enigmatic Edwardian: The Life of Reginald, 2nd Viscount Esher*, London: Sidgwick & Jackson, 1986, p. 301, quoted in David Loades, *Princes of Wales: Royal Heirs in Waiting*, Kew: The National Archives, 2008, p. 228.
59 Diana Vreeland, *DV*, New York: Knopf, 1984, quoted in Loades, *op. cit.*, p. 230.
60 HRH The Duke of Windsor, *A King's Story*, London: Cassell, 1951, pp. 254–5.
61 Quoted in Christopher Warwick, *Abdication*, London: Sidgwick & Jackson, 1986.
62 See Michael Bloch, *The Reign and Abdication of King Edward VIII*, London: Bantam Press, 1990.
63 *Time*, 9 November 1936.

64 Philip Ziegler, 'Churchill and the Monarchy, *History Today*, Vol. 43, 1 March 1993.

65 Lionel Logue papers, 28 October 1936.

66 William Shawcross, *Queen Elizabeth the Queen Mother: The Official Biography*, London: Macmillan, 2009, p. 376.

67 Rhodes James, *op. cit.*, p. 112.

68 *Ibid.*, p. 113.

69 Shawcross, *op. cit.*, p. 380.

70 Lionel Logue papers, 14 December 1936.

71 *Time*, 21 December 1936.

72 Lionel Logue papers.

73 Logue diary extracts: Lionel Logue papers.

74 *Sun*, 18 January 1938.

75 Wheeler-Bennett, *op. cit.*, p. 379.

76 *Ibid.*, p. 383.

77 *Ibid.*, p. 390.

78 *Ibid.*, p. 392.

79 *Ibid.*, p. 394.

80 *Ibid.*

81 Wheeler-Bennett, *op. cit.*, p. 405.

82 Shawcross, *op. cit.*, p. 488.

83 Wheeler-Bennett, *op. cit.*, p. 406.

84 *Ibid.*, p. 429.

85 *Ibid.*, p. 449.

86 *Ibid.*, p. 553.

87 Lionel Logue papers, 29 December 1943.

88 Wheeler-Bennett, *op. cit.*, p. 608.

89 *Ibid.*, p. 610.

90 Interview with the author, June 2010.

91 Lionel Logue papers, 10 December 1948.

92 *Daily Express*, 7 February 1952.

93 Wheeler-Bennett, *op. cit.*, p. 803.

94 *Times* obituary, 13 April 1953; response by J. M. Wimbusch, *The Times*, 17 April 1953.